Pelican Books
In the Servic

John Anthony Whitehead was born in Llanymynech,
Montgomeryshire, in 1926. He was educated at Oswestry
Boys' High School, Queen Mary College, London, and
the London Hospital. Before starting medical training
he spent some time in both the Royal Navy and the
Air Force. After qualifying at the London Hospital he
held various appointments in London and Shropshire
before going to Severalls Hospital, Colchester, in 1962.
It was during this period that he helped to open a
new general hospital psychiatric unit, and later developed
the psychogeriatric unit at Severalls Hospital. At the
moment he is Deputy Medical Director and Consultant
Psychiatrist at Prestwich Hospital, Manchester, and
Consultant Psychiatrist at Manchester Northern
Hospital. Dr Whitehead has published papers on general
hospital psychiatric units, mental illness in the elderly,
the organization of services for the elderly, and hospital
administration and communication. He has contributed
to books on psychogeriatrics and lectured on the
subject in the U.S.A. He is married, with three children,
and his interests include psychiatry, reading, writing and
living.

Anthony Whitehead

In the Service
of Old Age

The Welfare of
Psychogeriatric Patients

Penguin Books
Baltimore · Maryland

Penguin Books Ltd, Harmondsworth,
Middlesex, England
Penguin Books Inc., 7110 Ambassador Road
Baltimore, Maryland 21207, U.S.A.
Penguin Books Australia Ltd, Ringwood,
Victoria, Australia

First published 1970
Copyright © Anthony Whitehead, 1970

Made and printed in Great Britain by
Cox & Wyman Ltd,
London, Reading and Fakenham
Set in Linotype Times

'And that which should accompany old age,
As honour, love, obedience, troops of friends . . .'

Macbeth, v. iii

Contents

Foreword

It is as well for us that we cannot foresee our plight when our illusion of purpose vanishes as the winter of life sets in. For winter it is, relative to what has gone before, with its pride and loneliness, poverty and pain. Although some people are fortunate in being surrounded by friends, affection and property sufficient for their needs, many have little left. Once they retire income drops, the camaraderie of colleagues at work is lost, friends die off and changing fashions, tastes and attitudes engineer still further isolation and a sense of rejection by the world in general.

In this setting psychiatric illness characterized by depression, failing memory, clouded consciousness, agitation and irritability may blight existence and sour the last few precious months or years in this world.

The expectation of life at 65 is about thirteen years. Some thirteen per cent of the population is aged 65 years or more and of this number thirteen per cent will have a severe psychiatric disorder.

In this timely book Dr Whitehead has described our attempts at Severalls Hospital to develop an enlightened, hopeful and humane service for the elderly mentally-ill in a population of 750,000 people living in north-east Essex and part of east Hertfordshire. His purpose is to inform public opinion of what can be done and to stimulate self-scrutiny by authorities who should be doing more.

The competence, sincerity and humanity are as unmistakable in this excellent exposition as they are in the wards of the psychogeriatric service which he has developed. His style and his modesty may mislead readers as to the size of his contribution. I can only say that without him the success of the service and demonstration of what is possible within an existing budget would never have been achieved.

In congratulating Dr Whitehead on writing this book I would like to record my thanks to him publicly for the unfailing cooperation, loyalty and good companionship that he has always extended to me personally, as well as to the rest of our staff.

8 JUNE 1969   RUSSELL BARTON, M.B., M.R.C.P., D.P.M.

Physician Superintendent and
Consultant Psychiatrist,
Severalls Hospital, Colchester.
Consultant Psychiatrist,
Essex County Hospital, Colchester

Preface

In this book the problems presented by the elderly mentally-ill are discussed and some services available for their help and support are described. Particular reference is made to the comprehensive psychogeriatric service developed at Severalls Hospital, Colchester. This service, instituted and inspired by Doctor Russell Barton, has been established and expanded owing to the work of a number of doctors, nurses, social workers, administrators and ancillary staff. I have played a very small part in this work but a bigger one in writing the book.

Those involved have included: Doctors: P. K. Roy, S. M. Hanna, W. K. Marshall, E. J. Brown, S. Nirsimloo, S. B. Kazmi, I. Haider, D. J. Ball, D. J. Ellis, W. Allan, D. D. Thomson, E. N. Cheongve, T. R. Allan, D. Perara; Social Workers: Miss K. M. Jackson, Mrs J. V. Graham, Mrs A. M. Thurlow; Assistant Matrons: Miss C. M. Egan, Miss W. Hart-Davies, Mr T. Slack, Mr H. Robertson. Assistant Chief Male Nurse: Mr A. Walker; Sisters: E. Bowler, E. Raynor, V. Curtis, M. Garrod, P. Corner, M. Young, E. I. Smith; Charge Nurses: A. Nicholls, J. Dawson, J. H. Thomas, D. Stewart, C. Wood, W. Fox, A. Fairmanner, E. Loe, plus a large number of nurses and other workers, too numerous to mention. I hope they will excuse their names not being mentioned and realize this does not detract from the importance of their kindly contributions.

We do not claim originality and many of the things we have done we should like to do better, but we do believe we have tried.

I would particularly like to thank Doctor Russell Barton

PREFACE

for his inspiration and help with the minimum of interference, Doctor R. W. Revans for helping to clarify some of
my vague ideas, Mrs Barbara Robb for stimulating me to
write the book, the personnel of the various local-authority
health, welfare and ambulance departments for sympathetic
help and tolerance, a host of voluntary workers for all the
help they have given, all those who have helped with the
boarding-out scheme, the patients, their relatives and friends
and a number of people including Mr A. Adams, Mr W.
Kenny, Mrs J. Bryant, Miss D. Vernon, Mrs P. Dimond
and Mrs P. E. Balas who have given specific help with the
production of the manuscript.

SEPTEMBER 1969
J. A. WHITEHEAD
Prestwich Hospital,
Prestwich,
Manchester

1 | Introduction

The stimuli to write this book came from a number of sources. The work of many doctors, nurses, social workers, administrators and ancillary staff at Severalls had produced a service for the elderly mentally-ill which was not necessarily unique, but enlightened, human and hopeful. They had demonstrated what could be done for this group of patients, who are still often neglected and looked upon as beyond the help of modern medicine. There appeared to be a need to record this work as evidence of what can be done and to reinforce the pleas of many workers in the field of geriatrics and allied disciplines for a more positive, progressive and helpful approach to these patients. A number of papers had been published describing different facets of the work at Severalls, but these had appeared in a variety of journals in this country and the United States of America, not easily available to everyone interested in the problems of the elderly. This book is an amalgam of the information contained in these papers which give a fairly comprehensive account of the development and operation of the service.

The publication of *Sans Everything* (1967) brought to the attention of the public the plight of some elderly patients in some institutions. The picture painted may have been considered by some to be an exaggeration of the truth, with cruelty and malpractice too concentrated in place and time, but it was a reflection of reality. Anyone who has worked in a psychiatric or general hospital knows that cruelties sometimes occur. The commonest cause is ignorance, sadism playing only a minor role. It is hoped that the public will find in this account an example of what more enlightened hospitals are doing to help and support the elderly. It is also hoped that the staff of the few retarded authoritarian institutions still in existence in this country will be stimulated to look at themselves and see if they are doing all they can for the people in their care.

This is a description of the organization of a comprehensive service for the elderly psychiatric patient, developed on the principle that old people are healthier and happier if they can be supported out of hospital in their own homes, but should receive the best care available if admission is necessary. The pathological, clinical and therapeutic problems of mental and physical illness will not be considered, except very briefly where some knowledge of these subjects is necessary for the better understanding of the service. Readers interested in these subjects are referred to the books by Agate, Anderson, Comfort, Hazell, Howell, Irvine, Post and Stieglitz listed at the end of this chapter. The main themes will be: organization, communication, the development of a good therapeutic atmosphere, staff education and methods of stimulating staff interest and involvement.

The organization described can be used regardless of psychiatric orientation, being applicable to both a 'psychodynamic' and a 'physical' approach. It is also independent of narrow, medical divisions between physical and psychiatric illness. It could be used to deal with any old person in need of treatment, help or support.

What has been achieved so far at Severalls would appear to be the minimum necessary to help old people in need. Much more is required and is possible without great financial expenditure or increased staffing. It should be practicable to provide this immediate service in any part of the country.

Many people have contributed to the development of the Severalls unit, some being mentioned in the Preface. Their limited success has been due to a desire to solve problems, willingness to learn, and freedom to contribute without too much obstruction from authority. The organization and work discussed in this book is a record of what has been done; any opinions are my own, for which I take full responsibility.

References

Agate, J. N., *The Practice of Geriatrics,* Heinemann, 1967.
Anderson, W. F., *Practical Management of the Elderly,* Backwell, 1967.
Anderson, W. F., and Isaacs, B., *Current Achievements in Geriatrics,* Cassell, 1964.
Comfort, A., and Felstein, I., *The Process of Ageing,* Weidenfeld & Nicolson, 1965.
Hazell, K., *Social and Medical Problems of the Elderly,* Hutchinson, 1966.
Howell, T. H., *A Student's Guide to Geriatrics,* Staples, 1963.
Irvine, R. E., Bagnall, M. K., and Smith, B. J., *The Older Patient: An Introduction to Geriatrics,* English Universities Press, 1968.
Post, F., *Clinical Psychiatry of Late Life,* Pergamon Press, 1965.
Robb, Barbara, *Sans Everything: A Case to Answer,* presented on behalf of AEGIS, Nelson, 1967.
Stieglitz, E. J., *Geriatric Medicine,* Pitman Medical Publications, 1954.

2 | The Problem

The proportion of old people in the community is increasing and will continue to increase. Social and medical advances have not made people live longer but have made old age possible for a larger number. Coupled with this relative and absolute increase in the elderly population there has been a progressive tendency over the past hundred years for the old to become more isolated from their families and friends. Children move away because of their jobs, interests or from dissatisfaction with local conditions, while elderly parents are liable to migrate on retirement. Memories of childhood holidays and adult fantasies of peace and rejuvenation make the country and coast unrealistically attractive. Some find moving to a new home on retirement a pleasant experience and end their lives happily in a place where they have always wanted to live. Many, possibly the majority, realize that they have made a mistake when it is too late. They have moved from the familiar friend-populated place of their work to a new, strange world, new friendships are difficult to make, help is not available when needed and the winter, when it comes, appears a sad harbinger of death to come.

There is a belief, propagated by some politicians, that this is an affluent, over-pampered society in which everyone is feather-bedded by the Welfare State. This view has been maintained in spite of growing evidence, some anecdotal, but much scientific, that poverty, malnutrition, misery and neglect are still prevalent and possibly increasing. Two groups, children and the old, appear to be particularly affected and are the least able to expose their plight. The children are in the hands of their parents and the old do not complain because of pride, fear or apathy.

The increasing elderly population means that more old people are at risk of becoming physically or mentally ill. This risk is increased and complicated by poverty, malnutrition, poor living conditions and social isolation from their families and friends. The resulting mounting incidence of physical, psychological and social breakdown presents the health and welfare services with a caseload which some consider is beyond their capabilities. The Health Service, possibly one of the most enlightened and humane creations of the immediate post-war period, still struggles with a legacy of poor, ill-conceived properties called hospitals, a chronic deficiency of capital, and staff shortages. A common answer to these problems is to demand more money. Professor Millar has made a good case for the redistribution of Government spending (1967). Unfortunately, of all Government departments, the Ministry of Health is least pressed by the general public and pressure groups to spend more money. Most people tend not to worry about health unless they are ill, which is a sane attitude but not likely to lead to increased Government spending on health services.

Two other common approaches to the ills of the service are typified by the opinions of Enoch Powell and Arthur Seldon. Powell, in his book on medicine and politics (1966), discusses the problem pessimistically, finding faults and difficulties but hardly hinting at possible solutions. Seldon comments from the standpoint of conventional economics and has used the old chestnut about people needing to pay for a service directly if they are to appreciate it and use it properly (1967). Like Freud, he would appear to believe that the passage of money between patient and doctor makes for a good and satisfactory relationship. The same passage of money would also appear to be the suggested solution to the problems of a service caught up in the present technical revolution, yet held by the bonds of the past.

The Health Service is not a unified, rationally created organization equipped to deal with the overall problems of research, preventive medicine, diagnosis, treatment, rehabilitation and after-care for the disabled. It is a tripartite service and a compromise between past conflicting ideals and the present. The tripartite structure of general practitioner, hospital and Public Health sections is a product of its historical background and carries a number of serious disadvantages. Public Health, including community care service and associated welfare facilities, is controlled by local authorities and partially financed out of their funds, gleaned as rates from the local population. The general practitioner and hospital services are independently controlled and financed by the central government through executive councils and regional hospital boards. These financial arrangements lead to the drawing of sharp dividing lines between the functions of each service and the possibility of frequent demarcation disputes. The narrow, parochial views of some local authorities and regional hospital boards make cooperation between the different branches difficult, and highlight failings without contributing to their solution. In spite of fears of doing each other's work, duplication and overlap may occur, mainly owing to the poor communication that results from working in isolation. In areas where obsessional attention is paid to division of function the Health Service tends to operate inefficiently and patients usually suffer, many being sacrificed on the altar of administrative rigidity.

Hospital in-patient and welfare residential accommodation for old people is scarce, with gross over-crowding in many areas. Hospital doctors doing acute medical and surgical work are often loath to admit an old person to one of their beds because they are afraid the bed will become blocked if the patient cannot return home. They know that transfer to a geriatric bed may take months, during which time the patient can become a burden to nurses and not receive the special care and rehabilitation that the old require. Psychiatrists, more interested in younger patients, may also resist admitting old people and fail to organize a special psychogeriatric service.

Shortage of hospital and welfare home accommodation is not a matter of too few beds. Patients are not treated, rehabilitated, supported and nursed by bricks and beds. They need people with aptitude, sympathy and training. There is a world-wide shortage of medical, nursing and other personnel which affects even the two major powers, the U.S.S.R. and U.S.A. Neither planning nor financial encouragement would appear to solve this problem.

Over the past few years, a large body of knowledge has accumulated about the diseases, treatment and care of old people, with a better understanding of their medical, psychiatric and social problems. Unhappily, there is a technological gap between what is known and what is practised. No hospital uses all the knowledge available and some hospitals use relatively little. The care of the elderly tends to be unpopular. Doctors and nurses look upon geriatrics and psychogeriatrics as uninteresting and unrewarding, preferring to deal with younger patients. These attitudes are in part related to training in geriatrics which, until recently, had been nonexistent and still is generally inadequate.

Some medical schools have geriatric departments and there is a professor of geriatric medicine in Glasgow. In Oxford, post-graduate training is provided in both geriatrics and psychogeriatrics and the Maudsley, which provides excellent post-graduate training in psychiatry for a selective few, has a department of psychogeriatrics. Other centres provide training and experience in these branches of medicine, but too many graduates still have little knowledge or interest. Recently, two general practitioners in the North wished to take on a third partner. A young locum assistant working in the practice was offered the appointment, but said he would accept it only if they got rid of all patients on their list who were over the age of 65! He was not considered acceptable by the two partners. This may be an extreme case but many doctors can tell similar stories.

These are some of the problems affecting the support of old people in the community and their care and treatment in hospital. Some attempts at a solution have been very effective, others have tended to make the situation worse. A narrow view can lead to demands for more hospital and welfare home accommodation. If these are met, wards and homes are produced but cannot be staffed. Efforts to improve recruitment are made but when they fail they are sometimes used as an excuse for doing nothing more. The general shortage of money may lead to attempts at better utilization. Hospital staff are frequently urged to economize, but the usual result is some petty, irritating restriction such as charging staff for cups of traditionally free tea. The saving in actual money is usually very small, but the effect on morale can be devastating.

There are workable solutions for all the problems described and many hospitals and local authorities have made important contributions. Properly organized and coordinated, official and voluntary community care can do much to alleviate loneliness, isolation, malnutrition and the endogenous and reactive miseries that too often accompany old age. Effective community care relieves the strain on hospital beds and welfare accommodation, and indirectly disburdens the whole health service of some of its more general problems.

Much better use can be made of available resources. Perhaps a more rational and coordinated comprehensive health service will be developed as a result of present investigation and discussion. As a more immediate remedy, staff and services can be more effectively used by improving education and communication, encouraging social contact between all workers involved in the actual day-to-day work of the service and allowing everyone to make their best contributions. There is a vast wealth of knowledge, interest, enthusiasm and drive present in all grades of staff, but this is usually ignored and sometimes actively suppressed.

Matrons may claim that their hospitals are no longer authoritarian and psychiatrists talk of turning mental institutions into therapeutic communities, but most hospital staff remain status-conscious and Victorian in their ideas of staff management. Junior staff do what they are told and continue to follow archaic rituals that may have had some meaning in the past, but are now time-wasting, destructive of initiative and valueless. Porters may have ideas for improving their work, junior nurses may see what their seniors miss because of the blindness of familiarity, administrators may discover how clinical practice may be improved, but nothing happens. Time is wasted, the ideas of so-called inferiors are ignored, blindness continues and lay workers are afraid to trespass on the preserves of the self-protecting professionals.

In industry there is talk of worker participation in management and on the rare occasions when this has been tried it has worked. Staff relationships have improved, productivity has increased, with a dramatic reduction in disputes and strikes. Unfortunately, traditional management, jealous of its authority and position, afraid of change and grandiose in its self-delusions, resists these liberal innovations and usually destroys any faltering attempts made to implement them. Recent student protest has been aimed, at least in part, at obtaining student participation in university administration and teaching and has had some positive results. It does appear that this movement, which is really the natural development of modern concepts of democracy, is gaining some momentum. The Health Service needs both worker and patient participation if it is ever to overcome its present difficulties and develop into a humane public service. There are many obstructions to any move in this direction. Some doctors still feel superior to patients and other staff, delight in being individualistic and consider their orders should be followed without question. Nurses tend to be jealous of their not so recently acquired professional status and distrust anything that may deduct from their authority and established rights. Patients, in spite of increased public knowledge of medicine and the dissipation of medical magic, treat doctors and nurses as superior beings, rarely question what they are told and accept help like paupers. Progressive psychiatric hospitals are playing a part in making staff, patient and relative participation a reality. Good psychiatric hospitals encourage patients to play an active part in the running of their hospital, relatives are consulted as equals and all staff are allowed to contribute what they can. We are still a long way from real participation but if present improvements continue and are imitated, the psychiatric service in this country may yet become a model of enlightened administration. The obstructions to progress described can be overcome and, to a limited degree, have been overcome at Severalls. The result has been better treatment, a reduction in the number of in-patients and the creation of an enlightened service for the elderly.

References

Millar, Henry, 'In Sickness and in Health', *Encounter,* April 1967, pp. 10–21.
Powell, Enoch, *A New Look at Medicine and Politics,* Pitman Medical Publications, 1966.
Seldon, A., 'National or personal health service', *Lancet,* 25 March 1967, pp. 674–7.

3 | Old People and Institutions

In the last chapter, some of the problems set by the mounting elderly population were mentioned and briefly discussed. In this chapter, some specific problems will be considered in more detail, particularly the plight of old people in some hospitals, the place of the psychiatric hospital in geriatrics, and the effects of over-burdening hospital staff.

Long before *Sans Everything*, professional workers had published disturbing accounts of the plight of old people in hospitals and other institutions. Sheldon, in a report for the Birmingham Regional Hospital Board on hospital and welfare accommodation for old people in 1961, described accommodation that was poorly maintained, over-crowded, uncomfortable and depressing. Townsend in *The Last Refuge*, published in 1962, again described unsatisfactory physical conditions in many homes for the elderly and commented on the petty restrictions and authoritarianism still prevalent. He also pointed out that many residents need not be in such places but could have been supported in their own homes if the necessary effort had been made by the appropriate agencies.

Conditions in backward institutions are such that the most inexpert observer can see there is something wrong. Patients are herded together in old, bleak, neglected buildings with long dark wards, closely placed rows of beds, little furniture and frightening inactivity. Multiple regulations curtail the patients' freedom and reduce their contact with the outside world. They may be confined to the ward and allowed out only in large supervised groups. Privacy, usually valued by the elderly, is often nonexistent. Bathing is supervised and may take place in a communal bathroom. Visiting is restricted to a few hours per week and children are often prohibited. To visit some wards for the elderly is to visit the annexe to the mortuary. Rows of old people lie in bed with legs bent and muscles wasted by lack of use, eyes dull and vacant, waiting to die.

Three factors would appear to perpetuate these conditions:

   (i) Lack of satisfactorily motivated staff.

  (ii) Poorly trained staff, ignorant of modern geriatric practice and unaware of the basic emotional needs of the elderly.

 (iii) An authoritarian régime productive of petty restriction and staff fears.

There is a tendency for all three to occur together, the authoritarian régime possibly being the root cause.

A hospital run on authoritarian lines tends to be static. A system is laid down and adhered to with little chance of modification in spite of continuing progress in treatment and administration. It is usually inefficient because staff skills are not fully utilized and ideas are accepted only if they come from the top. Problems are solved by those in charge without adequate investigation and consultation. Rules are necessary to provide order, but once made, may be near impossible to change and in time become meaningless. Knowledge increases, situations vary and needs change, but the rules of an authoritarian institution, like the laws of an authoritarian country, become too firmly fixed to keep up with the present.

The authoritarian institution loses and fails to attract intelligent, better-trained staff, because they are unwilling to put up with the multiple restrictions and inhibiting atmosphere. To be even partially successful, an authoritarian system must have the conditions which existed in the old-time armed services. Here the rules could be enforced by the use of barbaric punishments, personnel were uneducated and escape was difficult and dangerous.

Authoritarianism spreads down from the top to all grades of staff. A 'pecking order' evolves, with staff passing the blame for anything that goes amiss. Everyone with the slightest authority develops a domineering attitude, coupled with a fear of those above. Assistant nurses, afraid of the ward sister, shout at and push patients who do not respond quickly to orders. An old lady in one psychiatric hospital used to call one particularly noisy and officious nurse 'Mrs Henhouse', neatly combining in this phrase the pecking-order concept and a description of the nurse's harsh, high-pitched voice. When things go wrong every effort is made to cover up the truth, facts are distorted, frank lies become commonplace, and true communication between staff is almost nonexistent. Patients are always seriously affected. Their freedom is liable to restriction, deviant behaviour is punished, ill-usage covered up, out-dated methods of treatment continued, and all the conditions productive of institutional neurosis fostered.

INSTITUTIONAL NEUROSIS

Institutional neurosis has been eloquently described by Russell Barton (1959). It is an illness of the inmates of institutions which is caused by the institution, and can occur in hospitals, prisons, concentration camps, monasteries or anywhere where people are removed from society and live in a rigid closed-off community. Sometimes it can develop in patients in their own homes, if the necessary conditions apply. Loss of contact with the outside world, and erosion of the personality by the overpowering control exerted by the institution are important factors in the production of this disease. The inmate becomes over-dependent, does what he is told because this is the only way to avoid trouble, loses initiative and interest and becomes one of a group of auto-matons. His appearance often demonstrates the effect the institution has had upon him: his face loses much of its expression, the head is held slightly bowed and the arms held semi-flexed with the hands closed. It has been claimed that these changes in personality and appearance are the end products of schizophrenia and, to a lesser extent, other psychoses. This is hardly likely to be true since the same picture is seen in patients who have had a large number of different illnesses and in some who have had no illness. Individuals vary in their response to incarceration in institutions; some remain relatively intact after years of confinement, while others succumb very quickly. The elderly seem to be particularly vulnerable and following admission to hospital soon come to look like their contemporaries admitted in early adulthood.

OVER-PROTECTION

Over-protection plays a part in the aetiology of institutional neurosis and in the creation of the bedridden ex-people described earlier in this chapter. Nurses tend to be preoccupied with the physical care of the elderly because they enjoy nursing, are trained to nurse and are often unaware of people's emotional needs, owing to one-sided, physically-biased instruction. Sometimes fear plays a part in creating an over-protective atmosphere. Traditionally, hospital staff fear trouble and believe any involvement with the coroner means serious trouble. Because of this, as well as for nobler reasons, abnormal efforts may be made to prevent patients injuring themselves. If an elderly patient falls in hospital and fractures a limb he might die and this might result in an inquest. To prevent this rather uncommon chain of events, any patients who are restless or unstable on their feet may be confined to bed. If the patient continues to be restless, the bed may be converted into a cage by the use of cot sides, or made up on the floor of a side room. Large doses of sedatives may also be tried to keep patients quiet, inactive and out of danger. Unfortunately, none of these manoeuvres works; confinement to bed during the day without occupation, conversation or entertainment increases restlessness and agitation, while sedatives, particularly the commonly used barbiturates, cause confusion and hallucinosis and increase erratic behaviour. The dangers of injury are increased, not diminished, because immobilization weakens muscles and makes bones more brittle, both of which are important precursors of fracture, while sedation and inactivity increase restlessness and confusion and diminish coordination. The patient, frightened and unsteady, climbs out of bed, trips, falls and sustains the fracture all this has been done to prevent. The disadvantages and dangers of confinement to bed have been known for years, yet patients are still put to bed unnecessarily and kept there longer than is required by their illness. In some hospitals, all patients admitted are automatically put to bed on arrival and kept there until they have been assessed. Assessment may only consist of a cursory physical examination, but the patient remains in bed for a week, by which time he may have become bed-fast and now require prolonged rehabilitation to undo the harm that has been done by hospitalization.

Confinement to bed has other serious consequences; bed sores may develop, incontinence of urine and faeces is likely to occur and a malignant form of institutional neurosis is almost inevitable. Nurses, unless they have been trained to consider the emotional and social needs of patients, are always liable to treat old people like babies, particularly if they are confined to bed. They feed them, wash them and too often purge them, but never treat them like adults. Their attitude is typified by expressions in common usage in geriatric wards. 'Which are the babies?' meaning, which are

being hand fed. 'Look after my babies'; 'Isn't she beautiful?' to describe a mumbling skeleton, caged in by cot sides
fastened to the bed. An ambivalent attitude is common so
that nurses invest a lot of time in giving careful physical care,
but are harsh in their emotional dealings and ignore the
patients' need self-respect: 'This is the wet and dirty
ward'; 'They are too filthy to have decent clothes'; 'You
filthy old thing, I shall smack you if you do that again.' Having reduced the patients to a state of helpless dependency,
the nurses criticize them for their regressed behaviour.

Over-protection can have ill-effects without the patient
being confined to bed. Patients who eat slowly or clumsily
may be hand fed by the nurse or ward aide. If they are
slow or uncertain about dressing themselves, this is done
for them and if they walk slowly, a wheel chair is used to
move them about the hospital or even the ward. Patients
who are unsteady and weak may be kept sitting in chairs and
never allowed to move about the ward. In this way, weak-
ness is increased and unsteadiness made more pronounced.

Over-protection extends beyond the care of the patient to
the care of their possessions. Following admission to some
hospitals, patients are stripped of their personal property,
including money, clothes, contents of pocket or handbag,
dentures, spectacles and hearing aids. Many reasons for
depriving patients of these articles are given by nurses, administrators and doctors. Property may be lost or damaged
and relatives will complain and public money will be wasted
on replacement or repair. Dentures get muddled and
patients may be given the wrong set, while hearing aids, not
only liable to damage, require adjusting, which takes up
valuable nursing time. Sometimes the only reason given is
that it is the custom of the hospital! Some of these excuses
are reasonable, others are not. Relatives do complain if
patients lose their possessions, but usually accept an adequate explanation. Spectacles and hearing aids may be

damaged but the cost of replacement or repair is insignificant against the importance of these aids to patients half-blinded and deaf because they have been confiscated.

Nursing time may be taken up sorting dentures and adjusting hearing aids, but it is well spent, in view of how much time is still wasted on traditional nursing rituals. Most articles, including hearing aids, spectacles, dentures, handbags, clothing, and a variety of personal knick-knacks, can be marked with the patient's name. It would seem inexcusable to deprive patients of means by which they eat, remain in contact with their environment and maintain a tenuous link with the world outside. It has been said that a rough method of measuring the efficiency of a geriatric ward is to count the number of patients out of bed during the day. Another is the ratio of personal belongings on or near the patients to the number in the sister's office or store.

OLD PEOPLE IN PSYCHIATRIC HOSPITALS

The lot of old people in some institutions has been described in rather depressing terms. What has been portrayed can apply to any establishment for the elderly. Many hospitals and homes are excellent but too many still have some, if not all, of the faults described, and psychiatric hospitals are no exception. Their place in the care of the old requires special mention, since this is a book about a service for the elderly based on a psychiatric hospital, and considerable concern has been expressed about admitting old people to such institutions. Reasons put forward for not admitting the elderly to psychiatric hospitals include: the fear patients have of this type of hospital, the stigma attached to admission, the poor quality of care they may receive and the isolation of many such hospitals. Similar reasons can be given for not admitting patients to many geriatric departments and welfare homes. These are often located in ex-Poor-Law institutions which engenders fears in old people, carry the same stigma for them, are often far from the patient's home and may be seriously under-staffed.

Elderly patients are admitted to psychiatric hospitals for a number of reasons. They may exhibit disturbed behaviour which makes admission inevitable, or they may suffer from a psychiatric illness that requires in-patient treatment. Other reasons may be less legitimate. In 1963 a number of correspondents to the *Lancet* discussed the demand for psychiatric beds and the problem of the elderly patient. Enoch claimed that psychiatric hospitals were being used as dumping grounds for old people (1963); many workers in these hospitals agree with this view, knowing that old people are admitted because no one else will have them. In some areas general hospitals will admit patients over 65 only if considerable pressure is used. Geriatric wards are over-crowded, and have mammoth waiting-lists and general physicians and surgeons are afraid that a 'valuable bed' will be blocked. General practitioners, in despair, turn to the psychiatric hospital, some modifying the picture of the illness a little to gain admission, over-stating the psychiatric symptoms and signs, while playing down the physical condition.

In many cases it may be difficult to decide which hospital should be responsible for the care of the patient. Unlike younger patients, old people tend to suffer from the effects of a number of different pathological processes and have a variety of symptoms and signs. Some diseases are inter-related, while others are independent of each other. Confusion, memory-defect and depression frequently complicate other illnesses. The patient may require help from general practitioner, geriatric physician, psychiatrist, local-authority health and welfare personnel and voluntary workers. The Health Service is more than tripartite when the elderly require help. The care of an old person in the community can present problems because so many different workers are involved. Some workers may disagree with each other over management and there can be disputes about who should do what. This is particularly likely to happen when the workers involved are paid from different sources. If admission to hospital or welfare home is considered necessary, different and more difficult problems occur because old people often have more than one disease at the same time and there may be symptoms of both physical and mental illness, whilst psychiatric symptoms are often the product of organic diseases. Due to these problems, the general practitioner may be unsure which hospital would be the best for the patient. When admission to a welfare home is considered because the patient is failing to care for himself, similar problems arise. The patient may be depressed or may have limited his activity because of an undiagnosed anaemia. There is always a shortage of geriatric and welfare places and the only accommodation available may be in the local psychiatric hospital, particularly if this hospital is an active, progressive establishment with a decreasing in-patient population.

A combined in-patient and community service for the old might be a solution to the difficulties. In this type of service, all beds for the elderly in a specific district would be under the control of one combined geriatric, psychogeriatric and welfare department. It would be difficult to establish, because of the present organization of services and resistance from the existing heads of each of the departments involved, since they would fear loss of autonomy and the dangers of subjugation to the new head of the combined department. It would have disadvantages, not the least of which would be an inhibition of varied development. At present, geriatric, psychogeriatric and welfare departments can develop in their own way, trying out new methods and techniques and generally contributing to our accumulation of knowledge of geriatric care. Combined units would have combined policies, so fewer different methods would be tried and fewer new techniques investigated. These difficulties and disadvantages are important but the old would gain more than they would lose from such a combined service.

Admission to a psychiatric hospital, provided it is the right hospital, can be a pleasant experience for a patient. Treatment and rehabilitation can be as effective as in a good geriatric unit even when the clinical condition is more 'physical' than psychiatric. Some progressive psychiatric hospitals offer patients better treatment than general hospitals because more attention is paid to the patients' emotional and social needs. This is not true of all mental hospitals, in some of which old people do not receive the care they deserve. A defeatist attitude may be taken to disease in this age group, with the result that little attempt is made to diagnose their illnesses accurately, or to treat, rehabilitate and return them to the community. Many physical diseases are curable, while mental illness does not necessarily carry a poor prognosis. Much can be done for depression, paranoid states, neurotic reactions and 'apparent' dementia. In the latter group, real dementia may be minimal, behaviour suggestive of this condition being due to unrecognized depression or other treatable illness. Many patients with true dementia can also be helped and successfully supported in the community.

The word *dementia* is used here to describe the deterioration in mental function that results from various types of brain injury. Damage to the brain is irreversible, but some of the clinical effects can be corrected and the picture is often complicated by other treatable conditions ranging from malnutrition to neurotic reactions. In the elderly, dementia is commonly due either to vascular degeneration interfering with the blood supply to the brain, or to senile degeneration of the brain substance itself. Its manifestations include memory defect, intellectual deterioration, uninhibited behaviour and loss of emotional control. In some cases, disturbances of speech occur, in the absence of serious deterioration elsewhere, so the patient, unable to express himself, appears much more demented than is the case.

Dementia can be mis-diagnosed or the degree over-estimated in a number of ways. The presence of speech defects can confuse the inexperienced doctor so that he may seriously misjudge the degree of actual dementia. Depression, malnutrition, physical disease and neurotic reactions may all confuse the doctor or nurse untutored in the care of the elderly. In many hospitals the diagnosis of dementia means that the patient will be treated as someone beyond help. He will be placed in a ward full of other demented patients and, except for being fed, washed and sedated, he will be ignored. The result, whatever the correct diagnosis, will be regression, dependence, loss of contact with reality and permanent hospitalization. Too often the apparent mental state of a patient at one point in time decides for ever his treatment and care. An example is the old man who becomes disturbed in the middle of the night because of some underlying physical illness. He is admitted to a psychiatric hospital far from his home where he is examined by a doctor who has been recently roused, bad-tempered, from his bed. The patient is asked a few questions rapidly about his name, age, address, the date, name of the hospital and perhaps the names of the Monarch, Prime Minister and a few world capitals in order to obtain a rough idea of his orientation and memory. The old man, ill, disturbed by the radical change of environment and a little upset by the attitude of the doctor, fails to answer some questions and answers others incorrectly. A diagnosis of dementia is made and this may decide treatment or lack of it until the patient dies in the institution. In fact his memory may be no worse than that of his contemporaries and his general knowledge may always have been limited.

The correct diagnosis, kindness and respect, adequate treatment and the provision of occupation and conversation would result in the old man recovering and returning home.

Failing memory, intellectual slowness and emotional instability, when present, should not mean that nothing can be done. Even patients with serious brain damage can have the quality of their lives improved by treatment of any associated agitation, depression, sleeplessness and incontinence. Many can be helped sufficiently to remain at home, or be discharged if in hospital.

Psychiatric hospitals are charged with the care of the elderly for four reasons.

(i) Some old people have to be admitted because of disturbed behaviour uncontrollable elsewhere.

(ii) Some require in-patient treatment such as electroconvulsive therapy, which is available only in a psychiatric hospital or unit.

(iii) Over-burdened in-patient facilities in geriatric and other general hospital departments apparently make it necessary for the psychiatric hospital to relieve some of the load by taking patients who are suitable for treatment in either geriatric or psychogeriatric units.

(iv) Long-stay psychiatric patients, legacies of the past and products of our present ignorance, grow old within the hospital, and become geriatric problems.

Since some old people necessarily come under psychiatric care, it is important that they should not be neglected. One approach to the problem is for each psychiatric hospital to open and develop a special psychogeriatric department. Staff interested in the elderly can then be recruited and trained and a comprehensive service, geared to the needs of the elderly inside and outside hospital, can be evolved.

THE ENLIGHTENED INSTITUTION

It is easy to find fault with the care given to old people in institutions, particularly when the conditions of work, shortage of staff and the technical difficulties involved are not appreciated and understood. Old people can be very self-centred, irritable and uncooperative. Treatment is often difficult and prolonged and requires staff with patience, understanding and an ability to remain interested in spite of knowing that the patient may die before the results of their efforts can be seen. The staff of most hospitals try to give their best, sometimes the results are impressive, but too often willingness is not combined with knowledge and freedom of action, so that care becomes unwittingly destructive, with the patient reduced to a bedridden, apathetic vegetable that is diligently washed, dressed, fed and ignored. Good care is easy to describe but difficult to practise.

There are many enlightened hospitals, hostels and welfare homes where an attempt is being made to employ a liberal policy and to utilize present knowledge to the full. Their success varies, but even the least successful is a very different place from the still extant old-type institutions. Patients appear alive, show interest in their surroundings, are cheerful and occupied. Staff aim at treating the old like adults and do not strip them of their personal possessions and their dignity. As far as possible, patients are allowed to have a say in what happens to them and it is realized that doctors and nurses do not necessarily know best. The therapeutic value of freedom is appreciated, privacy respected and contact with the outside world maintained by encouraging visits to the local town or village and allowing unrestricted visiting by relatives and friends, including children. Patients spend their own money on what they want and are not fed sweets and chocolates chosen by the staff. They are given a choice of food and not treated like

Victorian paupers. Every patient is encouraged to retain an interest in appearance by the provision of barber, hairdressing, manicure and other beauty-care facilities. Newspapers, magazines and books are provided in sufficient quantity and variety to satisfy everyone's reading needs, and the day is adequately filled with occupation and entertainment so that it is difficult to be bored, uninterested and withdrawn. A positive effort is made to make the old people feel wanted and useful, with something more to look forward to than the next meal, and death.

It may be claimed that all these aims are very commendable, provided the patients are reasonably active and not demented. It is a common belief that nothing can be done in the face of severe mental disability. It is easy to fall into this trap because personal anxieties can be damped down by the reassuring thought that no one can do anything for these patients except make them comfortable until death provides the final solution. A belief that mental patients are unaware of their surroundings is also reassuring when doubts arise about the physical condition of wards and departments. Many elderly psychiatric patients give an impression of remoteness from their environment when in fact there is no disturbance of contact. Examples are common in every progressive psychiatric hospital of patients who seem oblivious of what is happening regaining overt contact with reality when subjected to enlightened treatment. Some contact must always have been there, certainly enough to cause misery, if misery was at hand.

Following a prolonged programme of rehabilitation it is not an uncommon experience to see a ward full of incontinent, vacant-faced, hand-fed, immobilized and apparently severely demented patients become a community of interested, vocal, participating people. There are no satisfactory methods available for deciding how effective rehabilitation will be in a specific case. The effort must be made in all cases even if failure appears likely. This is one reason why the care and treatment of mentally ill old people is particularly difficult. Time, patience and energy may appear to be wasted, and staff are liable to give up, unless explanation, support and encouragement are available. Experienced, knowledgeable doctors and senior nurses are aware of these dangers, and must supply the support that is necessary for all grades of staff if an institution is to remain enlightened.

TOO MANY OLD PEOPLE IN HOSPITAL

A number of experts in different fields, dealing with the problems of old age, consider that there are many old people in hospitals and other institutions who should be in their own homes. Professor Townsend in sociology, and Dr Russell Barton in psychiatry, have frequently made this point. The majority of old people want to remain at home and many obviously do badly once removed from their familiar environment. The dangers and bad effects of ill-advised admission to hospital and welfare home will be discussed in more detail in later chapters. It will be shown that admission of an old person should always be viewed as a serious step and considered with the same care that a good surgeon takes when deciding on the advisability of a major operation.

Not only do many old people suffer when admitted to hospital, but many hospitals suffer by admitting too many old people. As mentioned in the previous chapter, demands for more geriatric and psychogeriatric beds are common. It is frequently claimed that another 50, 100, or 200 beds would solve the geriatric problems of a specific area. The bed is the magic symbol of need in both hospital and local authority welfare services. When beds are mentioned, buildings and services are included in the demand but the shortage of staff is forgotten. It may be possible to squeeze enough money out of a regional hospital board or county finance committee to build and equip another ward or hospital, but no board, however effective, or county council, however generous, can produce personnel if none are available. Recruitment drives, incentives and a more favourable labour market may result in a slight increase in staff numbers, but unless there are dramatic social and economic changes, the hospital and welfare services will remain short of staff, particularly for the care of in-patients and residents. As long as there is a shortage of personnel, there is a danger of patient care deteriorating. If a hospital operates fairly successfully with a certain number of in-patients, an increase of this number can, and usually does, result in a decline of care. If the increase is above a certain critical level for that hospital, the deterioration in care will accelerate. Overburdened staff lose heart, some leave, making the burden heavier, and finally only the basic physical needs of the patient can be catered for. Patients remain in hospital longer, more and more are there for life, beds are blocked and waiting lists snowball. The result is a further request to the authorities for more beds and the whirligig continues to revolve. Scientific evidence to substantiate these views is scant and confusing, but observations in a number of hospitals lend them support. Subjective impressions may be misleading, but no one can endorse overcrowding and the overburdening of staff involved in a difficult and trying task.

The support of more old people in their own homes should improve the standard of care in hospital. If the support in the home is adequate, many elderly people will end their lives in greater happiness and contentment than would be the case if admission to hospital were too freely advised. Adequate support at home requires community workers and staff for day hospitals and centres. Shortage of personnel would appear to work against both hospital and community care. In fact this is only partially true, since it is easier to recruit staff for community work and day hospitals than in-patient services. There are a number of possible reasons for this difference. In-patient care involves evening and night work which many people dislike. The real or imagined authoritarianism associated with working in a hospital also discourages recruits. Community work provides greater independence and freedom, while employment in a day hospital or centre does not involve evening or night work.

Experience at Severalls has shown that community support of more old people does relieve pressure on overworked in-patient staff and that recruitment of personnel for community work and the day hospital is relatively easier than for the in-patient service, and many old people's lives are improved by this emphasis on support at home.

References

Barton, Russell, *Institutional Neurosis,* John Wright, Bristol, 1966.
Enoch, M. D., 'Care of the Elderly Disturbed Patient', *Lancet,* 25 May 1963, p. 1,160.
Sheldon, J. H., *Report to the Birmingham Regional Hospital Board on its Geriatric Services*, published by the Birmingham Regional Hospital Board.
Townsend, R., *The Last Refuge,* Routledge & Kegan Paul, 1962.

4 | Severalls Hospital and its Psychogeriatric Unit

THE HOSPITAL

Severalls is located on the northern boundary of Colchester, a pleasant Essex town near the coast and within easy reach of London. The hospital was opened in 1913, having been built as a mental institution for the Essex County Council. It consisted of a centre complex of corridor-connected buildings for administrative services and wards, with the usual large central hall. Villa-type wards were scattered around the periphery and the whole was set in extensive high-fenced grounds, well-populated with trees and shrubs (Figure 1, pp. 42–3). All the buildings were one or two storeyed, the majority being the latter.

From 1913 until the inception of the National Health Service, Severalls was controlled by Essex County Council through a Committee of Management and would appear to have been very like other hospitals of its kind. A Medical Superintendent, all-powerful within the hospital but often rigidly controlled by the Management Committee and in fear of the Board of Control and the local coroner, was responsible for all the patients within the hospital. Other doctors working there were entirely under his orders and had no official responsibility for patients.

Until the Mental Treatment Act of 1930, only certified patients were admitted to mental hospitals of this type. This in itself had a profound effect on their administration and therapeutic climate. Patients with mental illness were recognized as being ill, but their compulsory admission and detention engendered a prison atmosphere of punishment, negation of human rights and degradation. High walls and railings, bare windows, locked doors, fenced-in exercise yards and padded rooms provided the prison environment. Within, patients were often treated like dangerous animals by part-trained staff armed with bunches of big, jangling keys, afraid and unaware of their charges' basic, emotional needs. When patients would not eat because of depression or paranoid fears of being poisoned, they were forcibly fed by two nurses. One held the patient with mouth open and the other shovelled in the food. Some patients, because of untreated mental illness coupled with boredom and frustration, occasionally tore their clothes. Instead of being provided with occupation, conversation and the chance to participate in ward activities, they were put in 'strong clothing' which is canvas dresses or suits, painful to wear and destructive to self-respect.

The introduction of voluntary status under the 1930 Act produced some improvement. Patients could now enter hospital for treatment without certification, which meant that less disturbed people were admitted, who, with their relatives, expected and asked for better and more humane treatment.

The hospital was responsible for admitting patients from most of Essex, but was not placed in an ideal geographical position for patients and relatives. At the time it was built, cheapness of land and administrative convenience were more important than consideration for 'lunatics' and their families. Since 1913 the catchment area has been changed, and now the hospital caters for a large area of Essex and east Hertfordshire (Figure 2, p. 45). The hospital is therefore even more remote from some of the area for which it is responsible, but this has been remedied in part by the opening of an associated psychiatric unit in a general hospital in Bishops Stortford on the Essex-Hertfordshire border (Barton, Herd, Whitehead and Brown, 1965).

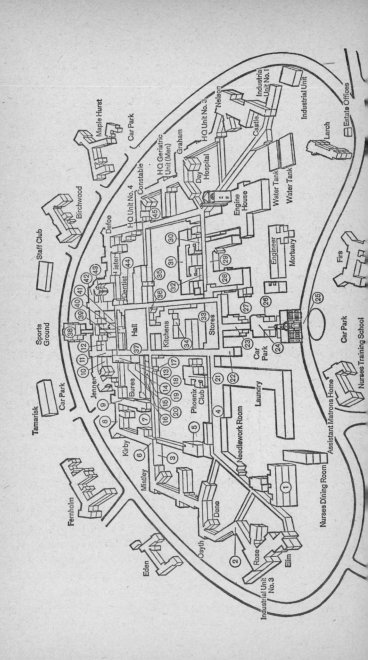

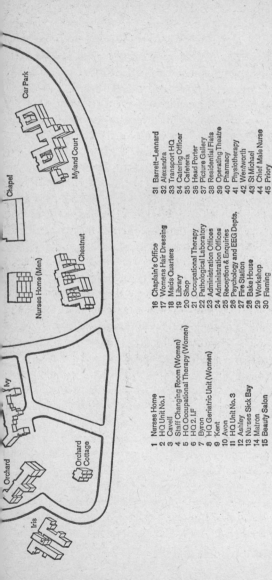

1 Nurses Home	**16** Chaplain's Office
2 HQ Unit No.1	**17** Womens Hair Dressing
3 Cavell	**18** Maids Quarters
4 Staff Changing Room (Women)	**19** Library
5 HQ Occupational Therapy (Women)	**20** Shop
6 HQ 2,I,F	**21** Occupational Therapy
7 Byron	**22** Pathological Laboratory
8 HQ Geriatric Unit (Women)	**23** Administration Offices
9 Kent	**24** Administration Offices
10 Avon	**25** Reception & Enquiries
11 HQ Unit No.3	**26** Psychology and EEG Depts.
12 Ashley	**27** Fire Station
13 Nurses Sick Bay	**28** Bake House
14 Matron	**29** Workshop
15 Beauty Salon	**30** Fleming

31 Barrett-Lennard
32 Alexandra
33 Transport HQ
34 Catering Officer
35 Cafeteria
36 Head Porter
37 Picture Gallery
38 Residential Flats
39 Operating Theatre
40 Pharmacy
41 Physiotherapy
42 Wentworth
43 St Michael
44 Chief Male Nurse
45 Priory

Figure 1. Plan of Severalls Hospital

In the Service of Old Age

The introduction of a National Health Service after the war resulted in mental hospitals being taken over by the Ministry of Health, and financed and controlled through various regional hospital boards. Improvement was now possible, but the most important Government contribution to better conditions in psychiatric hospitals was the Mental Health Act of 1959, which abolished the legal differentiation of general and psychiatric hospital, and ended certification as a status and as a procedure. Certification involved appearing before a Magistrate and the formal removal of certain human rights. Once certified, the patients became the responsibility of the mental hospital in which they were imprisoned. This in itself restricted plans for more enlightened treatment, since the hospital's first responsibility was to prevent the patient from escaping.

Patients could now enter psychiatric hospitals on an informal basis, that is, in the same way that admissions occur to general hospitals, without legal formality, and were now free to leave hospital whenever they wished. Under the previous Act, even voluntary patients had to sign an application for admission and could leave only if they gave three days' notice. After seventy years the mistakes of the restrictive Act of 1890 had been corrected. The 1959 Act still made provision for compulsory admission when necessary, but the power to admit compulsorily was removed from the hands of duly authorized officers and magistrates and given to doctors. Now, two doctors, one with special knowledge of psychiatry, had to see the patient before admission and sign the appropriate documents if compulsion was considered necessary. A system of appeal against compulsory detention was laid down to guard the freedom of the individual.

As a result of these administrative and legal changes,

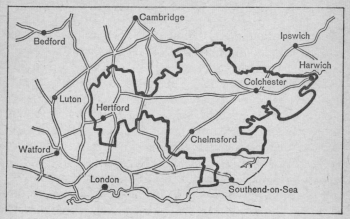

Figure 2. Severalls Catchment Area (area inside thick black lines). Scale: 1 inch = 16 miles

the introduction of new drugs, the revival of some older enlightened ideas of patient management including the provision of useful employment and leisure activities coupled with new concepts and a wave of better trained psychiatrists, a dramatic series of changes occurred in most psychiatric hospitals. The changes have not been universal and consistent because some senior staff are reactionary, like some members of every profession. Management committees fear change and some hospitals have failed to identify their problems and so have never solved them. No institution welcomes change and staff feel insecure when the reassuring familiar is threatened. As a result, they can easily block improvements by working in an obstructive way. For example, if wards are opened, patients may be allowed to wander away and in spite of unrestricted visiting, visitors may be discouraged from going to the hospital by the reception they receive from dissatisfied staff members. Severalls Hospital was able to change fairly successfully for a number of reasons. A new Physician-Superintendent had been appointed. Russell Barton had made a special study of institutions and had published his findings and recommendations in *Institutional Neurosis*. This set out in detail how mental hospitals could be improved, how resistance to advance could be identified and overcome, and how to involve the staff in making humane and successful psychiatric care a reality. Management did not fear change and a number of doctors, nurses and administrators were keen to see improvements carried out. New staff in all grades were appointed, who were selected because they were not wedded to the past, and a number made important, specific contributions, including the evolution of industrial therapy, a day hospital service and community care programmes. There was staff resistance to change, particularly among older members, but this was dealt with by free discussion and the involvement of groups of staff in special projects, such as the day hospital and industrial therapy. Some resistance occurred and continues, which is always likely to happen when change is a continuing process.

Severalls is not unique and there are hospitals scattered about the country that have developed in a similar way, some being more successful while others have advanced along slightly different lines. The changes described below occurred at Severalls but are an example of what every progressive hospital has done. Among other innovations, fences were removed, doors unlocked, patients allowed more freedom inside and outside the hospital, and relatives encouraged to visit at any time. Patients were allowed to see and visit the outside world, while the public were permitted to go in and see what was happening for themselves.

This enlargement of contact with the outside extended into all spheres of hospital activities. More interest and concern was shown for the lot of patients outside hospital, and more importance was placed on treating them in their own homes, so by-passing admission. It was at last realized that out-patient and after-care services were as vital as treatment in hospital. The number of out-patient clinics was increased and more use was made of 'domiciliary visits', where a hospital consultant, accompanied wherever possible by the family doctor, saw the patient in the home. Every effort was made to see most patients before they were admitted, a policy which prevents many unnecessary admissions. Mobile social workers were appointed to deal with patients' problems inside and outside hospital, and an increasing amount of social work was done by local authority workers. The duly authorized officers, successors to the Relieving Officers who dealt mainly with compulsory admissions under the old Mental Treatment Act, metamorphosed into Mental Welfare Officers, who were still involved with compulsory admissions, but now more concerned with the community support of patients. Local authorities also appointed psychiatric social workers, and the Welfare Department and National Assistance Board (now Ministry of Social Security) started to use field workers for the support of people at risk in the community. These developments necessitated greater cooperation between hospital and local authorities. Informal meetings were started between local authority and hospital personnel, and all outside workers dealing with patients in the community were invited to visit the hospital to discuss their problems and difficulties with hospital staff.

Mental hospitals tend to be places of morbid fascination and mystery to the general public. Strange, frightening beliefs are held about the inmates and what happens inside. To contribute to a better understanding of mental illness and to show that psychiatric patients are ordinary people who have become sick in a way different from the layman's concept of illness, but still sick, and not possessed or evil, the hospital staff gave many lectures to various organizations. These included Women's Institutes, the Townswomen's Guilds, Church organizations, luncheon clubs, professional bodies and schools. Organizations and individual members of the public were encouraged to visit the hospital and see for themselves what a modern psychiatric hospital is like.

This scheme of education for the public was coupled with a teaching programme within the hospital. Lectures, clinical meetings and symposia were held for hospital doctors, nurses and ancillary staff. Courses were organized for general practitioners, health visitors, staff from other hospitals, social workers and the clergy. Other hospitals were visited to help staff expand their view of the hospital service, learn new techniques and perhaps obtain more insight into their own failings by studying the successes and failures of others.

BUILDING IMPROVEMENTS

Severalls, like most mental hospitals, had been starved of money for years with a resulting deterioration in the physical condition of wards and departments which had never been ideal. The wards were too big, poorly decorated, and inadequately furnished and equipped. In 1960, an extensive programme of ward reorganization was started. Where possible, large wards were split up into smaller units. Many wards were two storeyed with sleeping accommodation above and dining and day facilities below. This was changed so that most became self-contained on one floor, ground-floor wards being reserved for the elderly.

One large, two-storeyed villa was converted into a modern admission unit for men and women. It included a mother and baby unit, occupational therapy, art and music departments and a unit for electro-convulsive therapy.

The latter served the whole hospital and dealt with both in-patients, day patients and out-patients.

The hospital shop was enlarged, the range of its stock increased and a café opened. The shop was allowed to sell matches to patients. This was looked upon as a dangerous revolutionary step by older staff members who had fantasies of fires breaking out all over the hospital. This did not happen. When matches are prohibited and smoking re-stricted to short supervised periods, patients conceal matches or lighters and smoke in secret. These conditions are more likely to lead to fires than to prevent them.

Long-stay patients tend to neglect their personal appear-ance, and new patients have often lost interest because of their illness. A beauty salon and barber's shop were opened to discourage these negative attitudes and to improve the appearance and morale of patients. One member of the nursing staff specialized in the removal of facial hair and made an important contribution towards improving the appearance of older ladies in the hospital.

Physical improvements to the hospital have included much more than has been described and are continuing. This account is an illustration of what has been done and a demonstration of the ways in which some psychiatric hos-pitals are developing.

THE UNIT SYSTEM

The majority of mental hospitals are large and over-crowded. Severalls at one time accommodated over 2,000 patients, having been built to deal with 1,800. The numbers have now been reduced to 1,130 in spite of catering for an increasing population and more people asking for help. This has been due to a number of factors, most of which will be described in this account of the psychogeriatric unit, but which are in fact applicable to the whole hospital and the majority of other progressive hospitals in this country. The development of out-patient facilities, more use of home visits, day care and the coordination and augmentation of community care services has meant that more patients can be treated without being admitted, and many in-patients can be discharged because of the support and help now available outside hospital. Within the hospital, improved treatment and more active, intelligent rehabilitation programmes have resulted in quicker recovery from illness and the rescue of long-stay patients, previously abandoned to perpetual inactivity and hopeless, permanent residency. The reasons why some hospitals have been more successful than others have already been mentioned, and without doubt, any hospital that has failed to reduce the number of in-patients has failed in its duty to the public and should seriously and conscientiously examine itself, identify its faults and blocks to progress and attempt to correct them.

There has been considerable discussion about the ideal size of psychiatric and general hospitals and there appear to be as many different opinions as there are experts. Economically and administratively, size must be important, but it is doubtful if anyone knows enough about the subject to be dogmatic. Good patient care and treatment does not depend upon the overall physical size of the institution. It depends on the closeness of the hospital to the community it serves and on the organization within and without. Patients are treated by a consultant, his junior doctors and a group of nurses and ancillary workers. If the group of people involved in treatment make up a well integrated group and can be kept together, the therapeutic advantages of a small hospital can be transferred to a hospital of any size. A unit system was devised at Severalls which gave each consultant a group of neighbouring wards and beds in the admission unit and specialist wards. Each unit had a staff group consisting of one or two junior doctors, assistant matron, assistant chief male nurse, social worker, secretary, ward nurses and occupational therapists. Except for student nurses who have to move from ward to ward to gain the necessary experience, members of the staff were kept together on each unit for as long as possible. In this way, mutual understanding developed and patients came to know and to have confidence in the staff involved in their therapy.

There is a movement to incorporate psychiatric services in the general hospital complex and ultimately to close the existing psychiatric hospitals. There are many advantages to this plan but at present psychiatric hospitals must continue to play a major part in caring for the mentally ill. The advantages of general hospital units are that they do not have the stigma of mental hospitals, are in closer contact with other branches of medicine and are more likely to develop active, progressive treatment and rehabilitation programmes, since they are all relatively new and tend to be nearer the population they serve. Some of these advantages can be obtained by psychiatric hospitals if they convert some of their wards into a general hospital unit, catering for the normal community. Severalls, like a psychiatric hospital in the North, has started to do this. It has a surgical unit which is associated with the local general hospital and which deals with the usual range of general surgical cases from the community. The work of this unit has caused a considerable reduction in the number on the waiting list of one of the consultant surgeons at the local general hospital. Plans have been made to increase the size of the surgical unit and add a medical unit, accommodation becoming available as the number of psychiatric patients in the hospital decreases. The introduction of general surgery into the hospital has helped to change the attitude of the local population. They are coming to look upon it as a hospital and not as a lunatic asylum.

In the Service of Old Age

The introduction of a new range of drugs for anxiety, depression, mania and schizophrenia, and the use of electro-convulsive therapy and leucotomy, together with a whole range of treatments for neurosis, have obviously been important in helping patients with psychiatric illness and changing the pattern of their care. The development and use of these treatments has coincided with other important changes. The open door policy, with greater freedom for patients and a more permissive, tolerant atmosphere, has gradually removed a number of anti-therapeutic attitudes and procedures which destroyed the personality and reduced the chances of recovery. The increased use of occupational therapy and, perhaps more important, the development of industrial therapy, have also helped to rehabilitate and return to the community many long-stay patients and have prevented the development of the 'chronic sick' syndrome in many new ones.

The new treatments have been used extensively at Severalls with results similar to those in many other hospitals. Industrial therapy has played a large part in the new régime. The importance of useful, meaningful, interesting employment has been emphasized by some people involved in the treatment of the mentally ill for very many years. Nineteenth-century lunatic asylums employed patients in many activities, including work in the institution's laundry and farm, though it does appear that this was more for economy than treatment of the patient. During the past twenty years, enlightened psychiatric hospitals have done a lot to provide useful work that rehabilitates and prepares patients for life in the outside world. Bristol has a very large industrial therapy organization where patients can do a variety of jobs for which they are paid and which prepare them successfully for normal employment in the community. Industrial therapy at Severalls was initiated and evolved due to the drive, knowledge and involvement of the Physician Superintendent, the late Chief Male Nurse, Mr Knifton, a Senior Registrar, Dr Morgan who now runs a very successful rehabilitation hospital in the Midlands, and a number of doctors and nurses who followed them. There are now two main factories producing saleable articles ranging from dolls' houses to dressing gowns. Other units produce boxes, concrete blocks and package nuts, bolts, screws and nails. A household management unit offers rehabilitation for the housewife, with facilities for meal planning, cooking, washing and ironing.

Independence has become a virtue not a sin, and patients have been encouraged to take a more active role in the running of the hospital. Some wards hold regular patients' meetings where opinions can be freely expressed. These may be combined or associated with staff meetings and range from a forum for the airing of views and complaints to more formal therapeutic sessions. Patients are expected to make decisions both about themselves and the ward organization, to ask questions and disagree with staff. They are guided, not ordered, and in every respect treated like adults, and not like refractory children who have to be controlled like the unfortunate inmates of puritanical reformatories.

THE PSYCHOGERIATRIC UNIT

Most of this chapter has been taken up with a general description of Severalls and the services it now provides. The psychogeriatric unit is one unit in the hospital. Description here will be limited to a general outline since a more detailed account will be given in the chapters that follow.

The unit was established in 1961, four male (145 beds) and six female (229 beds) ground-floor wards being set aside for this purpose. Patients were admitted to the unit from two main sources – from within the hospital and from the community which was the Severalls catchment area. Severalls provides psychiatric services for a major part of Essex and east Hertfordshire (Figure 2, p. 45). The population of this area in 1961 was 647,000 and had increased to 714,000 by 1965. The patients from within the hospital had either grown old within the institution or had been admitted by a consultant to a bed in his unit as an emergency.

From the beginning, the unit operated on the principle that old people should be maintained in their own homes for as long as possible. Admission to hospital, when necessary, should be only for a short period, unless longer and permanent admission was inevitable. Provided the home is kept intact the condition of the majority of patients admitted can be improved sufficiently to enable them to return and be maintained in the community. Some, of course, may be too ill ever to leave but the number that fall into this category should be very small if the hospital is providing an efficient service in the wards and in the community. To make this possible two social workers were employed to work both within the hospital and within the community. Nursing staff started to assist in community work outside hospital, visiting patients in their homes, arranging community support and counselling both patients and relatives. A 'month-in/month-out' system was established, by which the care of more disabled patients could be shared between the hospital and family. The patient spends a month in hospital followed by a month at home and then a further month in hospital and this is continued as long as necessary. The families obtain relief and the patients are not cut off from the community and know that when a month is over they will return home. A day hospital was opened since day care is an essential part of any service for the elderly. The usual range of treatments was provided including drug therapy, group and individual psychotherapy, physiotherapy, occupational and industrial therapy, social rehabilitation, electro-convulsive therapy and habit training for incontinence. The latter consists of the re-education by the nursing staff of patients who are incontinent of urine, faeces or both by taking them to the lavatory at regular intervals. This at first keeps them clean and later, in many cases, results in the patient becoming continent without assistance from the staff, because a habit has become re-established.

In December 1963 the unit was reorganized. A planned admission procedure was established, the 'month-in/month-out' system was modified and extended, day care was made available to a larger number of patients, a 'boarding-out' scheme was introduced and plans for an emergency service were considered. Provisions were made for admitting married couples to the same side room when both needed in-patient care or when it was considered by the medical, nursing or social work staff that separation was damaging or unkind and the partner wished to be with the patient.

During the next few months other schemes were started. Weekly review conferences were held, attended by the unit's medical staff, senior nurses and social workers. All patients who had been admitted for a limited period were reviewed, progress was checked and treatment and supportive plans modified or executed. Regular meetings between hospital staff and local health and welfare workers were established as one method of improving relationships and communication. At these meetings mutual problems were discussed and methods of providing coordinate care explored. Relatives were involved in therapy by holding regular relatives' conferences in the hospital, to which all relatives and any other interested members of the community were invited.

The staff of the unit are supplied with a leaflet describing its general policy of preventing the unnecessary admission of old people to hospitals, their support in the community and the methods available for making this policy work.

With the leaflet is a timetable of weekly and occasional meetings. Examples of these documents are shown in the Appendix. The actual content of these documents and the routine has varied throughout the life of the unit, owing to the continuous changes that have occurred and should occur in a progressive service. Many such documents have been issued because of these changes; the ones reproduced in the Appendix are examples.

Many psychiatric hospitals are becoming overcrowded with elderly patients. Both hospital staff and the public complain, yet very little is done. Experience at Severalls would suggest that there are solutions to this problem which reduce in-patient populations and benefit the elderly. Between 1961 and 1967 the number of in-patient beds in the psychogeriatric unit was reduced by 97 from 145 male and 229 female to 107 male and 170 female. One female ward was converted to a day hospital and a male ward was taken over by another unit. All of the beds were never filled. This occurred in spite of an increasing caseload and increasing demands for help. The decrease in the number of in-patients would appear to have benefited patients, staff and community. Care in hospital has improved and an increasing concern with community support has brought help to larger numbers than would have been possible if in-patient treatment was all that was available. Community care in general will be described in the next chapter and this will be followed by more detailed accounts of specific community projects, the organization of the in-patient unit and communication between hospital and community.

References

Barton, Russell, Herd, J. A., Whitehead, J. A., and Brown, E., 'A New Psychiatric Unit for a Mixed Urban and Rural Population', *The Medical Officer*, 1 January 1965, pp. 3–5.
Mental Health Act, 1959, H.M.S.O., London.

5 | Community Care

The majority of old people do not like being removed from their own homes. They value independence, freedom and the presence of familiar faces and objects. Some rather unscientific observations and other more accurate work by a number of investigators has shown that the old in fact do badly when removed from their familiar environment and are usually happier and healthier if they can remain in their own homes. There are some exceptions, particularly among ex-service men and retired old-type domestic servants, who appear to prefer communal life and may be glad to enter an institution in old age.

The opinion of those who say they prefer to remain at home and to die there is of some value, particularly when applied to themselves. Illness may seriously interfere with judgement, but most elderly patients who resist admission when confused resist even more strongly when they are well. A proportion of elderly persons admitted as patients are very much upset by the experience, never recover and end their lives in apathetic misery. Too large a number after admission to hospital develop new illnesses which appear to be related to the change of environment, and even a short period in hospital may have catastrophic results on health and social competence. Many elderly people are supported in the community by a delicate web of help provided by neighbours, friends and regular visitors such as postmen, milkmen and rent collectors. Admission, if clumsily effected, may permanently break this web, making resettlement difficult or impossible. A comparison of the appearance and behaviour of day patients with in-patients suffering from similar clinical conditions also supports the hypothesis that old people are better out of hospital. Day patients tend to be happier, more active, better dressed, more interested in what is happening and more communicative.

Studies of the ill effects of admission to hospital or transfer from one institution to another have all tended to confirm these impressions (Camargo and Preston 1945, Kay, Norris and Post 1956, Litin 1956, Whittier and Williams 1956, Rang 1957, Lieberman 1961, Newman 1962, Aldrich and Mendkoff 1963, Kent 1963, Reichel 1965, Rosin and Boyd 1966). Some of these workers have shown that elderly patients in hospital often develop new illnesses which are apparently unrelated to the disease that brought them into hospital and seem to be due to the change of environment. Others have examined the effects of transferring a group of old people from one old people's home to another. This move took place because of a rebuilding programme and not as an experiment. They found that this group of people tended to develop more illnesses and died earlier than would have been expected if they had not been moved.

This combination of opinion, observation, impression and investigation supports a policy of keeping old people in their own homes. The Health Service in the past concentrated its activities on developing and improving hospitals at the expense of community care and there is still too much emphasis on in-patient services. Removal to hospital or welfare home is sometimes necessary but possibly the majority of admissions could be prevented and many more patients discharged if community care was fully developed.

Old people are always in danger of removal from their homes. Their precarious situation has been well depicted in a cartoon (Figure 3, p. 60) by Dr Russell Barton (1965). Doctors and social workers may apply their own middle-class standards to a home and find it wanting. Ignoring the emotional needs of the old person and the dangers of admission, they then press for institutional care. Pressure for admission may come from relatives, friends or neighbours who have become over-anxious, sometimes as a result of guilt. Occasionally, motivation is more questionable. The house is wanted by a relative, neighbour or property developer and the old person is standing in the way. Community care, if adequate and well organized, can provide an answer to some of these dangers. Support may relieve pressure and anxieties and sometimes community workers are able to prevent the unscrupulous from getting their way.

THE GROWTH OF COMMUNITY CARE

Plato recommended family care and a human approach towards the mentally ill in his *Republic*. A few in every age may have held these views but little was done to implement them until the middle of this century. There have been notable exceptions such as the Gheel community in Belgium, which has provided foster-home care since the Middle Ages. In wealthy families care at home has usually been possible, but the poor, dependent on society for support, were offered only the workhouse, lunatic asylum, house of correction or prison.

During the nineteenth century, in spite of the *laissez-faire* policy of succeeding governments, enlightened public pressure produced a series of important reforms indicative of concern for the individual. Progress towards a more humanitarian society has continued because this pressure has been sustained. The introduction of a National Health Service, the National Assistance Act of 1946 and the Mental Health Act of 1959 have had important effects on the treatment of the mentally-ill. Limited community care services, mainly for the physically-ill, had been available for many years. Voluntary organizations, churches and individuals have

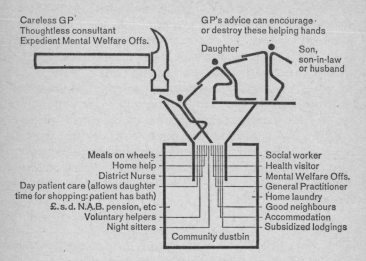

Figure 3. The factors that help a patient to float in a community, and those that tend to push him under, into an institution

always done work that can be described as community care, and some hospitals developed their own after-care. A famous example is the Robert Jones and Agnes Hunt Orthopaedic Hospital, Oswestry, which has always had an after-care service for cripples. District nurses have provided nursing care in the home since 1859. In that year William Rathbone, a Liverpool merchant, started a system of home nursing which soon spread to the whole country. District voluntary committees coordinated by the Queen's Institute of District Nurses were responsible for this service until it was taken over by the local authorities after the Second World War.

These provisions for the physically-ill rarely extended to those with mental sickness. In-patient care in an asylum was usually all that was available until after 1946. There were no out-patient clinics except in the larger cities and even there they dealt only with limited groups of patients and were unevenly distributed. During the post-war period, as a result of legislation, public opinion and individual interest and effort, a complex of community services for treatment, rehabilitation and support have been developed. Some of these services can be used for patients with any type of illness, while others have tended to be more specific. The background to community care, its development and present structure are described by Professor Lady Gertrude Williams (1967), A. F. Young and E. T. Ashton (1956) and M. Penelope Hall (1963).

COMMUNITY CARE FOR THE ELDERLY

Almost all community organizations can play a part in supporting old people in their own homes. The possible services available are illustrated in Figure 4 (p. 62). The two-way arrows in the diagram are intended to illustrate the potential for the free exchange of information and help. It will be seen that certain services have to be provided but others are optional or depend on the interests of voluntary organizations. The result is considerable variation in the provision of community care throughout the country. In some areas services may not exist or only partially function while others have the maximum amount of help possible. Services that have to be provided may be inadequate and optional ones nonexistent. A long list of community care organizations can give a false impression of the actual service provided. Home helps may be scarce and their use limited to certain patient-groups such as maternity, and sick young mothers with children. 'Meals-on-wheels', if functioning, may supply meals on only two days a week. If an old person has difficulty with cooking or preparing food because

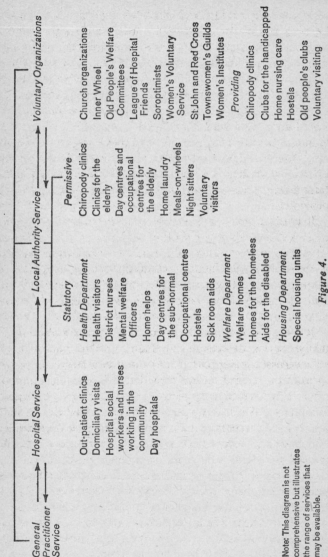

COMMUNITY CARE

General Practitioner Service → Hospital Service → Local Authority Service → Voluntary Organizations

Hospital Service

Out-patient clinics
Domiciliary visits
Hospital social
workers and nurses
working in the
community
Day hospitals

Local Authority Service

Statutory

Health Department
Health visitors
District nurses
Mental welfare
Officers
Home helps
Day centres for
the sub-normal
Occupational centres
Hostels
Sick room aids

Welfare Department
Welfare homes
Homes for the homeless
Aids for the disabled

Housing Department
Special housing units

Permissive

Chiropody clinics
Clinics for the
elderly
Day centres and
occupational
centres for
the elderly
Home laundry
Meals-on-wheels
Night sitters
Voluntary
visitors

Voluntary Organizations

Church organizations
Inner Wheel
Old People's Welfare
Committees
League of Hospital
Friends
Soroptimists
Women's Voluntary
Service
St John and Red Cross
Townswomen's Guilds
Women's Institutes

Providing

Chiropody clinics
Clubs for the handicapped
Home nursing care
Hostels
Old people's clubs
Voluntary visiting

Figure 4.

Note: This diagram is not
comprehensive but illustrates
the range of services that
may be available.

of psychiatric or physical disability, two meals a week is hardly enough. An investigation into the dietary of elderly women living alone in 1965 indicated that the meals provided by the 'meals-on-wheels' service were sometimes inadequate, low in Vitamin C and unappetizing because of the delay between cooking and eating. The report of this investigation suggested that meals should be provided at least four times a week. A number of workers involved with community care consider that the meals supplied in some areas are too high in carbohydrate, too low in protein and often unpalatable. It is claimed that because of the latter fault a number of old people feed their pets with the meals provided.

It is often said, particularly by hospital staff, that community care consists of visiting patients and writing down what is wrong but doing nothing about it. Unfortunately this is sometimes true. Some community social workers look upon physical work such as lighting a fire or preparing an urgently needed meal as degrading to the dignity of their office.

It is easy to find fault with community care and there are many obvious defects and inadequacies, but many patients are successfully supported and there is a steady improvement in the overall service provided. The usual explanation for slow and not rapid improvement is shortage of personnel and money. This may be partially true, but there is considerable overlap of services and an uneconomic use of resources. A case was discovered in one part of the country where one young family was visited by representatives of fifteen different agencies. All gave advice, usually conflicting, but little practical help was offered except the provision of a daily home help which was not needed. In the same area it was impossible to obtain a home help, even one day a week, for an old man living alone and completely dependent on neighbours.

In some areas of the country, close relationships have been developed between hospitals and community services, with benefit to both. In these areas – of which Nottingham, Croydon and Salford are examples – effective community care is becoming a reality.

SEVERALLS AND COMMUNITY CARE

Community care for the elderly has been briefly described and discussed in general terms. No particular distinction has been made between the needs of old people with physical and those with psychiatric illness. In fact there is no place for distinction, since the needs and problems of support in the community are similar, whatever clinical divisions are made. An attempt has been made at Severalls to devise a co-ordinated community care service for elderly psychiatric patients. Sharp lines are not drawn between different illnesses and some patients with few psychiatric symptoms are treated and supported.

From the beginning, hospital staff have been actively engaged in community work. Social workers and nurses work in the community, and medical staff spend a proportion of their time visiting patients in their homes, meeting other field workers and coordinating supportive services. Over a period a service has developed that dovetails with local authority and voluntary community programmes. The unit's contribution can be considered under five headings. This makes description easier, but it should be remembered that all types of therapeutic and supportive care are interdependent and tend to be ineffective in isolation. The five convenient headings are: Hospital Staff Working in the Community, Coordination of Community Services, Day Care, The Emergency Service, and Boarding Out. Only the first two will be considered here: the others are dealt with in detail in later chapters.

HOSPITAL STAFF WORKING IN THE COMMUNITY

Hospital staff frequently resist attempts to admit old people but do not offer any assistance to their support at home. This is an approach that may keep a few patients out of hospital but does little to solve problems and usually generates community ill-will. Local-authority workers and individual and organized volunteers do a lot to support the elderly in the community and do not appreciate obstruction to the admission of patients with whom they can no longer cope. The special skills of hospital personnel may make further support possible, but for this to happen these skilled personnel have to be available in the community. When hospital doctors, nurses and social workers spend time working outside the hospital, existing community services benefit from the extra help and specialized knowledge made available, while the hospital staff gain insight into the problems of patients and their families. Closer contact between hospital and community workers also provides an opportunity for better communication and possibly improves mutual understanding.

One unforeseen consequence of the unit staff concerning themselves with community work has been a significant reduction in the number of compulsory admissions. In 1965 a number of letters appeared in the *Lancet* on the subject of the compulsory admission of patients to psychiatric hospitals and units. Some psychiatrists including Enoch and Barker suggested that Section 29 of the Mental Health Act 1959 was often being used when patients were willing to come into hospital without compulsion on a so-called 'informal' basis (1965).

Section 29 provides for the compulsory admission of a patient with psychiatric illness to hospital in an emergency. The order requires the signature of only one doctor, usually the patient's general practitioner, and is effective for three days. Following admission to hospital the order can be rescinded, allowed to lapse at the end of three days, or extended, depending on the views and judgement of the responsible hospital doctor. Other sections of the Act deal with the compulsory admission of patients who are not emergencies. In these cases two doctors are required to see the patients before admission and to sign documents to the effect that compulsory admission is necessary. One of these doctors must have special experience of psychiatry and is usually the consultant who will treat the patient in hospital. In some areas the second doctor is a general practitioner considered to have special knowledge of psychiatry, but this rather unsatisfactory practice is becoming less common.

Experience at Severalls and the associated general hospital unit in Bishop's Stortford confirmed Enoch and Barker's findings. An example of the misuse of compulsion occurred in the Bishop's Stortford unit in 1962. A Polynesian with hypomania was accepted as an emergency under Section 29. During the interview following admission he said he had been trying to get into hospital for three days. He had been a patient in a London psychiatric hospital in the past and, realizing he was becoming ill again, he had asked to be readmitted. This was refused because he had no doctor's letter. He tried two other hospitals with the same result. By this time he was more severely ill and decided to undress in the street to attract attention to himself. Compulsory admission quickly followed without the doctor or mental welfare officer involved considering asking the patient if he wished to enter hospital of his own accord.

Similar if less dramatic examples were considered to be commonplace when the subject of unnecessary compulsory admission was discussed at staff meetings in the hospital. The psychogeriatric unit staff carried out an investigation into the use of compulsion in their unit and discovered that few compulsory admissions occurred in spite of many patients being referred with the claim that it would be necessary. Only three to four such admissions occurred each year. The judicious use of mental welfare officer, hospital social worker, or nurse, depending on the attitude and needs of the patient, appeared to have been one factor in producing this low incidence compared with other units and hospitals. Other possible factors were the staff's dislike of compulsion, a willingness to spend time in persuading patients to co-operate, the use of the emergency service and the overall provision of a variety of supports in the community. The last two factors made possible the support of patients at home when they refused to come into hospital.

A system had evolved as a result of the emotionally therapeutic atmosphere in the unit which treated all patients as individuals with rights and opinions. When a patient was referred for admission by a general practitioner who considered compulsion would be necessary, a home visit was made by either a doctor, social worker, nurse or combination of these, depending on availability of staff and the situation described by the patient's doctor. Sometimes it would be found that the patient did not need to come into hospital and could be treated at home, sometimes day hospital care was necessary and occasionally admission was considered advisable. In every case the patient was seen by a unit doctor either in the home or day hospital before a final decision was made.

In almost every case visited, kindness and explanation resulted in the patient accepting either help at home, day care or admission to hospital. Sometimes more than one visit was necessary before a satisfactory relationship could be developed between the staff and patient. In some cases a social worker or nurse would have to collect the patient and bring him to the day hospital on a number of days before he would come in the normal ambulance. Patients who were known to the unit, having been in-patients or day patients on a previous occasion, were usually visited by someone who knew them and had developed a good relationship with them in the past. When it appeared that the patient would respond best to a particular individual he was dealt with by the appropriate member of staff. For example, a retired hospital sister with strong ideas about the status and importance of nurses developed a paranoid illness, refused all help offered by the general practitioner and would not see a unit doctor when he visited her. A sister from the hospital was asked to visit her and it was suggested it would be best if she wore her full uniform for the visit. As a result the old lady came into hospital willingly, cooperated in treatment and was soon well enough to return home.

The low incidence of compulsory admission was not the result of a conscious effort to produce impressive statistics. The unit staff were not aware that compulsory admissions were so few until the admission details were analysed. Anti-authoritarian teaching and staff efforts to provide a humane service for the elderly would appear to have created the necessary atmosphere and conditions in which compulsion becomes a rarity.

Hospital staff, like any large group of people, consists of some who are hard and unfeeling, some who are very tender-hearted and a majority who are neither. This majority will tend to behave in a manner conditioned by the institution. If there is rigid authoritarian discipline and patients are allowed to suffer indignities such as being deprived of possessions and restricted in their activities because of the system, staff will tend to be harsh and unfeeling with both their colleagues and their patients. Compulsion and punishment will be used because they naturally fit into the general pattern. Patients react to this situation by becoming cowed, rebellious, or disciplined but dissatisfied and liable to angry outbursts. Violence breeds violence and fights, attacks on staff and staff cruelties to patients are likely to occur. If the same institution with the same nurses and ancillary staff and patients becomes more liberal because of the introduction of a progressive policy from above, and senior staff show more kindness and understanding, dramatic changes occur. In time the whole atmosphere alters, violence and cruelty disappear, locked doors become unnecessary and compulsion is a forgotten relic of the past.

COORDINATION OF COMMUNITY SERVICES

An important function of the unit social workers is to supply information on community services and coordinate these services for patients. This applies equally to patients being discharged and patients for whom admission can be prevented. The social workers know what services are available in different parts of the catchment area and are able to arrange the maximum possible support for each patient. This is coordination of community services at the simplest but often the most difficult level. Any experienced worker in this field of social work knows that what is available in any area depends on good communication and good relationships. Formal requests for home helps or 'meals-on-wheels' may be met with kindly rejection. Closer contact with the appropriate organizer and a little sympathetic understanding often produce help where none apparently existed before.

Contact between hospital, local authority and voluntary worker is maintained by a variety of informal meetings. The communication at regular meetings is augmented by the normal personal contacts which occur when people are allowed to work freely together. A telephone call or discussion over a cup of tea in the day hospital can achieve more, more rapidly and with more mutual understanding, than pages of formal, stilted correspondence.

An attempt has been made to remedy the misuse of

manpower owing to overlap and duplication of services, by making one worker responsible for the organization and support for each patient. This may be a hospital social worker, nurse, local-authority mental welfare officer, psychiatric social worker or welfare department field worker. Some duplication still occurs but is becoming rarer and never involves more than two agencies.

THE EFFECTIVENESS OF COMMUNITY CARE

The effectiveness of any service that treats and supports people is hard to assess because of the number of factors involved and the difficulties of measurement. Not only must the patients be considered but also their inter-action with the family and the rest of the community. This is a subject that will be discussed again in other chapters dealing with the particular community services provided by the unit.

At Severalls it has been possible to integrate hospital-based community care with local-authority and voluntary services. Coordination of all the agencies involved, and increased cooperation and understanding appear to have benefited patients, community workers and hospital staff. This is an impression based on a number of observations and supported by work in other areas.

The in-patient and community services continue to function fairly efficiently in spite of a considerable increase in referrals and in the total number of patients supported inside and outside hospital. More patients and families are helped than would have been possible if in-patient care only were available. Many patients have come under care and have been helped who would never have been seen if nothing but incarceration in hospital were available. Support for these views has been provided by the work of Peter Sainsbury and his co-workers.

Sainsbury and his colleagues have carried out a number of investigations into a psychiatric community care programme in West Sussex, comparing this service, based on a day hospital, with a more conventional hospital-orientated service which admitted the majority of patients referred. In one study of elderly patients (Sainsbury, Costain and Grad, 1965) it was shown that more patients were referred to the community-care-biased service and many fewer were admitted to hospital. There appeared to be little difference between the two groups of patients as far as diagnostic categories and severity of symptoms were concerned, but the community service appeared to recruit more of the under-privileged and lonely. A psychiatric service that is concerned with community support is liable to attract larger numbers of clients because people are more willing to seek help if they know it can be provided outside hospital. The psychiatrist and his staff working in the community become known and information about the service they provide spreads. Patients ask their general practitioner to refer them for psychiatric advice and the general practitioner is more willing to do this because he knows effective community care is being provided and has seen it work in his practice. Hospital-orientated services are usually remote, tend to be feared and are often ignored by general practitioner, patient and family unless the patient has to be admitted to hospital or relatives cannot cope any longer. The under-privileged and lonely are more likely to be helped by a community-biased service because the workers in this type of service are usually more aware of the community's needs and make efforts to meet them. On the whole, patients dealt with by the community service spent shorter periods in hospital when hospital care was temporarily necessary, but those with more severe disorders stayed in relatively longer than similar patients admitted to the hospital-biased service. This may have occurred because patients admitted when effective community support was available were likely to be more severely disturbed than those admitted to hospital when little else was provided.

Findings at Severalls have been similar except for the last result. Patients with severe symptoms have tended to remain in hospital for only short periods, while the most severely disabled have been maintained by an organized system of recurrent short admissions (variants of the month-in/month-out system). In the same paper Sainsbury and his co-workers put forward the hypothesis that lonely old people who retire to resort towns are in more danger of developing mental illness than their peers who remain in familiar surroundings. Part of the Severalls catchment area has a number of coastal towns popular as places of retirement. The large number of patients referred from these towns supports Sainsbury's suggestions.

Grad and Sainsbury, in a later study (1968), have examined the effects of community care on the family. A cohort of patients treated by the two different services was followed up over two years, and the effects on the patients' families were measured. When the total number of patients involved was considered, regardless of age or diagnostic category, it appeared that the community service which favoured extra-mural care left the patients' families more heavily burdened. This did not hold good, however, when the families who had been the most severely burdened at referral were considered separately. These families were helped equally in both services, even though significantly few patients were admitted by the community-biased service. In the same way, families of all patients over 65 were not adversely affected to a significantly greater extent in the community care service. It appeared that it was the treatment of the younger, mainly psychoneurotic patients which accounted for the overall difference in burden between the two services, suggesting that for these persons, in-patient treatment would be the service of choice for the families concerned.

The evidence available appears to support the use of community care for the elderly. Patients prefer to remain out of hospital, more patients and families can be helped and the burden on the family is still relieved. Community support for the elderly in its present form is relatively new and is continually changing. In progressive areas hospital and community workers try out new and modify old services in an attempt to provide better care for the patient. It would appear important that more studies of the effectiveness of these services should be undertaken. Factual objective studies will help future planning and should increase the chance of community care becoming a well established method of helping people without removing them from society.

References

Aldrich, C. K., Mendkoff, E., 'Relocation of the Aged and Disabled: a Mortality Study', *Journal of American Geriatric Society*, March 1963, pp. 185–94.

Barton, Russell, 'The Inter-Dependence of Hospital, G.P. and Community Care', *Medical World*, May 1965, pp. 1–6.

Camargo, O., and Preston, G. H., 'What Happens to Patients who are Hospitalized for the First Time when Over 65 Years of Age?' *American Journal of Psychiatry*, September 1945, pp. 168–73.

Enoch, M. D., and Barker, J. C., 'Misuse of Section 29', *Lancet*, 3 April 1965, p. 760.

Enoch, M. D., and Barker, J. C., 'Misuse of Section 29', *Lancet*, 29 May 1965, p. 1,161.

Grad, J., and Sainsbury, P., 'The Effects that Patients have on their Families in a Community Care and a Control Psychiatric Service – a Two-Year Follow-Up', *British Journal of Psychiatry*, March 1968, pp. 265–78.

Hall, M. Penelope, *The Social Services of Modern England*, 6th Edition, Routledge and Kegan Paul, 1963.

In the Service of Old Age

Kay, D. W. K., Norris, V., and Post, F., 'Prognosis in Psychiatric Disorders of the Elderly. An Attempt to Define Indicators of Early Death and Early Recovery', *Journal of Mental Science,* January 1956, pp. 129–40.

Kent, E. A., 'Rôle of Admission Stress in Adaptation of Older Persons in Institutions', *Geriatrics,* February 1963, pp. 133–8.

Lieberman, M. A., 'Relationship of Mortality Rates to Entrance to a Home for the Aged', *Geriatrics,* October 1961, pp. 515–19.

Litin, E. M., 'Mental Reaction to Trauma and Hospitalization in the Aged', *Journal of the American Medical Association,* 22 December 1956, pp. 1,522–4.

Newman, J. L., 'Old Folk in Wet Beds', *British Medical Journal,* 30 June 1962, pp. 1,824–7.

Rang M., 'Incidence of Complications among Elderly Hospital Patients', *Lancet,* 23 February 1957, pp. 401–2.

Reichel, W., 'Complications in the Care of Five Hundred Elderly Hospitalized Patients', *Journal of the American Geriatric Society,* November 1965, pp. 973–81.

Report of an Investigation into the Dietary of Elderly Women Living Alone, King Edward Hospital Fund for London, 1965.

Rosin, A. J., and Boyd, R. V., 'Complications of Illness in Geriatric Patients in Hospital', *Journal of Chronic Disease,* March 1966, pp. 307–13.

Sainsbury, P., Costain, W. R., and Grad, J., 'The Effects of Community Service on the Referral and Admission Rates of Elderly Psychiatric Patients', *Psychiatric Disorders of the Aged,* Report on a Symposium held by the World Psychiatric Association, London 1965, pp. 23–37.

Whittier, J. R., and Williams, D., 'The Coincidence and Constancy of Mortality Figures for Aged Psychotic Patients Admitted to State Hospitals', *Journal of Nervous and Mental Disease,* December 1956, pp. 618–20.

Williams, Professor Lady Gertrude, *The Coming of the Welfare State,* Allen & Unwin, 1967.

Young, A. F., and Ashton, E. T., *British Social Work in the 19th Century,* Routledge & Kegan Paul, 1956.

6 | Day Care

It can be seen from the last chapter that the successful support of patients in the community depends on the development of an interlocking complex of different services. Day care in its various forms is an important part of any community care programme for the elderly but must fit in to the general pattern of support. Day care at Severalls has evolved as part of a network of in-patient and community services. The day hospital not only helps with community care but acts as a bridge between hospital and the world outside.

THE DEVELOPMENT OF DAY CARE

Occupational centres for the sub-normal, opened in 1914, were the beginning of our present concept of day care. The first day hospitals for psychiatric patients were introduced in the U.S.S.R. between the Wars. During the Second World War a geriatric day centre was opened in New York. The first psychiatric day centre in Britain was opened in London in 1946 by Bierer – the same year that Cameron started day care in Montreal. Since 1946 day hospitals and centres for all types of patients have mushroomed in Britain. Farndale in 1959 visited sixty-five day hospitals and centres and mentioned 350 occupational centres (1961). The number has increased considerably since this investigation.

The terms 'occupational centre', 'day centre' and 'day hospital' do not have an accurate definition. On the whole, day centres and occupational centres are run by local authorities or voluntary organizations, while day hospitals are the responsibility of the hospital service. Day hospitals are manned by doctors, nurses and ancillary staff offering care similar to an in-patient service without bed and breakfast. They provide the usual in-patient treatments, supervision of any necessary drug taking, occupation, food, company and perhaps a feeling of belonging. Day and occupational centres do not usually provide medical and nursing care, and are more concerned with occupation, entertainment, food and social activity.

The idea of a psychiatric day hospital was to provide something between in-patient and traditional out-patient treatment. They could act as a stepping-stone between hospital and community, making discharge easier and smoother, and prevent the admission of certain patients, so protecting them from the possible ill-effects of in-patient care. Another important function was to blur the sharp dividing line between the patient who could be treated as an out-patient and those who required institutional care.

Day hospitals have assumed various mantles. Some are neurosis centres, treating patients not normally admitted to traditional mental hospitals. Others act as halfway houses for patients who have recovered from a psychosis in hospital but still need some security and support before they can fully return to a normal life in the community. Some have become psychogeriatric day units, while geriatric hospitals have developed their own type of day hospitals which sometimes cater for patients with psychiatric symptoms (Cosin, 1956), but usually confine their activities to the treatment of physical illness and infirmity. In spite of the increase in the number of day hospitals and centres, their distribution is uneven and in many parts of the country day care is either not provided or the provision is for such small numbers that it has little effect. Possibly the least well provided for tend to be the elderly mentally-ill. The majority of geriatric day hospitals and local-authority day centres will not accept old people with psychiatric symptoms and very few mental hospitals make any provision for them. For example, one large city in the North with a population of over half a million has no special day hospital facilities for the elderly mentally-ill and many other large areas of population are similarly placed.

ADVANTAGES AND DISADVANTAGES OF DAY CARE

Day care can prevent admission while providing help for patient, relatives and friends. The patient is not cut off from the community, dangers of rejection are reduced, while skilled treatment and rehabilitation normally available to in-patients only is provided. Day hospitals can be sited near the community they serve and act as a centre of out-patient and community support. When this happens coordination of services is easier and community and hospital workers are brought into closer contact with each other, so reducing misunderstandings and making real two-way communication possible.

There are disadvantages. Patients can become dependent on the day hospital and this can be as severe as the dependence developed by long-stay patients of institutions. Transportation can present problems for old people. Public transport is rarely suitable for this group of patients, and in rural areas is normally inadequate, even if the patient is sufficiently mobile and competent to make use of it. This means that the ambulance service must be used. If the number of day patients is large, the ambulance service may become overburdened and unable to collect and return on time. This can be upsetting to the patient and may generate conflict and ill-feeling between the hospital and the ambulance authority.

Attendance at a day hospital may result in unnecessary admission. A patient may be referred because the general practitioner considers that company and a little treatment may help, but does not believe that in-patient care is necessary. Hospital doctors and nurses, seeing the patient in isolation, become over-anxious, build up fantasies of what might happen to the old person on returning home and admit him or her as an antidote to their own anxieties.

Financial considerations cannot be dismissed as immaterial to patient care. Day care is no cheaper than in-patient care, but the burden is shared between the hospital and local authority. What the hospital saves is spent by the ambulance service providing transport, so cost is neither an advantage nor a disadvantage unless a narrow view of hospital cost alone is taken.

THE EVOLUTION OF DAY CARE AT SEVERALLS

When the psychogeriatric unit was opened in 1961, a day hospital was included in the unit. An existing male ward with some in-patients was used because no other accommodation was available at that time. Owing to staffing difficulties, only male patients were accepted. Medical and nursing staff showed little interest, some nurses being actively opposed to the project, with the result that few patients were referred for day care and those that were tended to feel unwelcome. The reasons for this opposition are difficult to analyse. Overtly it was claimed that the day hospital was doing the work of the local authority, which was considered to be unfair to the hospital, and covered up the inadequacies of local authority community care. Conflicts with local-authority workers, unrealistic fears of redundancy and a general resistance to change all possibly played a part in producing this attitude. Resistance to change was made more acute by the variety of changes occurring in the hospital at this time. Most of these changes, particularly unrestricted visiting, more freedom for patients and the encouragement of people to visit the hospital, tended to break down the barriers between the hospital and the community. Day care was seen as another breach in the wall. Many nurses, especially the older ones, may have felt threatened, insecure and unprotected, since taking down fences not only opened up the world to the patients but let the world see what was happening inside.

In 1963 with the reorganization of the unit, day patients were accepted on two female wards. Later one female ward, emptied of in-patients, became a mixed day hospital. An increase in the number of day patients made it necessary in 1965 to move the day hospital to a larger ward that had become available because of the reduction in the number of in-patients. In 1967, 250 patients were attending, the daily average being between 130 and 170. This increase occurred because of a policy change in the unit and, more important, because of increased interest in day care. Medical staff started to think of day care when seeing out-patients, nurses interested in the project were recruited, while nurses already employed were encouraged to think about and discuss this method of treatment and support. As the day hospital flourished, further interest was generated. When it was seen to work, without threat to nurse or harm to patient, more staff members were converted and often the most resistant became the most enthusiastic.

ORGANIZATION

The organization of the day hospital at Severalls has been concisely described by Haider (1967). The building finally used had been a typical mental hospital ward, remaining bleak, poorly decorated, under-furnished, over-occupied and locked, while other wards had been transformed. Emptying it of in-patients not only made more day hospital accommodation available, but removed the last ghetto. The dormitory became an occupational and entertainment centre, side rooms became offices, treatment and examination rooms, while the old dining-room and sitting-room continued to fulfil these functions. Curtains, paint and non-institutional furniture changed the physical conditions. The atmosphere was changed by staff and patients.

The nursing staff are mainly part time, working either mornings, afternoons or for the total period the service is available (from 9 a.m. to 5 p.m., five days per week). The majority would not be interested in working in the hospital if this type of work had not been available. The sister in charge was a retired ward sister who returned to work because of her interest in day care. No extra medical staff were employed. Day care is a normal part of the service offered by the unit and is not looked upon as something outside the usual work and responsibility of the unit's medical staff. Since it is an integral part of the service, all the facilities of the hospital are available to day patients. These include industrial and occupational therapy, various entertainments, individual and group psychotherapy, a household management unit, hairdressing, chiropody, bathing, physiotherapy, pathological and radiological services, electroplexy and the hospital shop and library. These services are put in no special order, so that one may not be considered more important than another. The list is not comprehensive but illustrates one important advantage of a day unit being part of a hospital. The physically separate day hospital could provide these services only at great expense both in money and personnel. A more important advantage of this type of unit is the increased possibility of continuity of care. A patient is able to move from out-patient to day patient to in-patient and back again and still retain contact with some staff members. Out-patients are mentioned because the day hospital also took on the functions of an out-patient department. This has made it possible for patients to spend the day in hospital, have a meal and bath if necessary and be observed and investigated more thoroughly than would be possible in a conventional out-patient department. Patients tend to find this a pleasanter experience than attending the more usual out-patient clinic.

The majority of patients are transported to and from the hospital by local authority ambulances. They usually arrive between 9.30 a.m. and 10.30 a.m., returning home between 3.30 p.m. and 5 p.m. On rare occasions, because of pressure on the ambulance service, some patients may arrive later or have to return home after 5 p.m.

On arrival they are given tea. Newcomers are introduced to staff and patients and shown around the unit. The morning is spent in various activities and in treatment. Lunch is at twelve noon and is supplied free of charge. The afternoon is spent either resting, or engaged in industrial and occupational therapy or the various entertainments provided, including occasional lectures and demonstrations by guest speakers. Tea is provided before departure.

New patients are seen and examined by a unit doctor on arrival. Care has to be taken not to frighten the patient away. Some patients are only briefly examined on their first visit, more intensive investigation being postponed until they have settled in and become accustomed to environment and staff. Nurses often want to bath new patients almost before they have taken off their hats. This is discouraged because some old people are afraid of hospital-type bathing and may be put off by this insistence on obsessional cleanliness. After a few attendances they may ask for a bath or be persuaded to have one without the appearance of authoritarianism.

All patients are seen daily by the doctor during his informal round and private interviews take place at varied intervals depending on the needs and problems of the patients. General medical as well as psychiatric care is provided. Patients are not expected to go to their own general practitioner with physical ailments, but can do so if they wish.

Rigid rules, dignified as ethics, rarely help patients and do little to improve the patient's concept of the doctor.

There is only one day hospital at Severalls and this is for elderly patients. Young day patients are catered for in the in-patient wards and other departments. A few young patients work in the day hospital as helpers. In this way a service geared to elderly needs is maintained without complete segregation by age. Diagnostic categories include the whole range of psychiatric illness, the majority having some type of organic brain disease. The age range is from 58 to 96, with women outnumbering men by three to one.

It has been claimed that old people dislike travelling and are upset by long ambulance journeys. The disruption of daily routine resulting from attending a day hospital or centre has also been considered a serious disadvantage of this type of care. Patients come from a radius of twenty-five miles to the Severalls unit and few complain of the journey, in spite of criticism being encouraged. A very small number do object to travelling and some suffer from motion sickness. In these cases they are either treated at home or admitted, depending on their illness and the social problems associated with it. Some patients enjoy the ambulance journey more than the session in the day hospital. This would appear to be either a tribute to the therapeutic atmosphere in the ambulance or a criticism of the service provided by the hospital. One woman always complained if the ambulance failed to pick her up on its way to an outlying village, because she liked the trip into the country and felt she had been cheated if she was carried directly from home to hospital.

Patients who are being discharged from in-patient to day patient care are encouraged to attend the day hospital for a few days while still in-patients. In this way the change-over is made more smoothly and failure to attend as a day patient becomes less of a risk. If patients are admitted who have previously attended the day unit, they visit this unit for part of each day during their in-patient stay. This makes admission more acceptable and makes continuity of care a reality.

Patients are expected to play an active part in running the service. Weekly patient/staff meetings are held in which free discussion is fostered, and initiative on the part of the patients is encouraged. Patients are asked for their views and criticisms and their assistance is sought in devising methods of improving the facilities and producing new types of occupation and entertainment. Many changes have taken place because of patients' suggestions, including the provision of more occupational and industrial therapy and visits, talks and demonstrations by experts on various domestic science subjects. The successful treatment of a patient has often been the result of the efforts of other patients who by their kindness, explanations and practical help with accommodation and the provision of interest and company outside the hospital have done more than the professional staff in the rehabilitative process.

TRANSPORT

The success of a day hospital for elderly patients must depend on the cooperation and goodwill of the ambulance service, since most patients require an ambulance because of their disability and the general inadequacy of public transport. The cooperation of the ambulance service is not simply a matter of public servants doing their job. Unless the personnel, both senior and junior, feel involved, many difficulties may arise. There are always reasons why patients cannot be collected and returned on time, and rules, real or conveniently self-created, to prevent people from doing what they do not want to do. Excuses include the pressure of more important work, such as accidents or medical and surgical emergency, and rules that prevent ambulance crews entering houses and persuading people to come to hospital or waiting while they get dressed. All these and many more factors may make the running of a day hospital difficult and unsatisfactory.

Fortunately, these problems have not occurred at Severalls. One reason has been the quality of ambulance service personnel. Another has been the effort made to involve them in the project. Senior officers visit the unit frequently and are invited to all social functions organized there. The problems of the unit are discussed informally and openly. Ambulance crews are made welcome, supplied with cups of tea and are encouraged to take part in social activities. An effort is made to keep a two-way flow of information, ideas and criticisms. This is not done by official letter, circular or news sheet but by personal contact in kitchen, day room and roadway. The result has been goodwill, understanding and a desire to help. The practical effect has been a willingness to do much more than is normally expected of an ambulance crew.

Two problems did arise soon after the day hospital was started. Patients were sometimes not ready when the ambulance called, or refused to come, and others had to return to a cold, empty house in the evenings. Often ambulance crews were able to deal with these problems by ignoring regulations, but too often this was not possible.

These problems were solved by arranging with the ambulance service for a nurse to go out with ambulances which had problem patients on their list. The number of these cases is small at any one time, so this has not presented a serious staffing problem. With the development of the service, ambulance crews have tended to do more unofficial work, reducing the need for a nurse to accompany them.

In many hospitals, complaints about the ambulance service are common and ambulance crews often complain about hospital personnel. This would appear to be the result of isolation and the use of official channels. A chat over a cup of tea in the kitchen between a nurse or doctor and an ambulance crew member can solve more problems and generate more mutual understanding than hours of discussion by a committee or a working party. There is no need for procedural gymnastics and self-glorification in the kitchen.

RELATIONS WITH THE COMMUNITY

A day hospital can play a unique part in closing the gap between community and hospital. Patients bring the outside world into the hospital and take out ideas and impressions that can benefit or damage the hospital's image. If the day unit is run on liberal principles, relatives, friends and community workers should have free access and play a similar role in improving the community's concept of the hospital and the hospital's concept of the community.

Relatives welcome day care. The idea that families want to dump their elderly relatives in institutions for life is misleading. A few have this attitude, but many make considerable sacrifices to keep the old person at home. The majority who seek help have withstood difficulties, inconvenience and often misery for years. An old person who is confused, restless at night and of uncertain temper can place great strain on a family, and love tends to have a limit. Relief from some of the burden is often all that is required. Owing to ignorance or incorrect advice given by doctors or community workers, relatives may believe that institutional care is the only help available. When day care is discussed, many families are relieved to find that help without the trauma of permanent removal is possible. The family is freed during the day. Treatment may improve behaviour and ensure restful nights, while association with the hospital helps relatives to deal with their problems because they no longer feel alone. Regular relatives' conferences augment these more informal contacts and provide a milieu in which problems that arise with old people in the home can be talked out with others in a similar situation.

The whole range of community workers has become involved in day care at Severalls. Psychiatric social workers, mental welfare officers, health visitors, district nurses and home helps often stimulate general practitioners to refer cases. New patients are frequently brought in by community workers who have dealt with them before referral. Hospital staff have been all but forced into relationships with outside organizations because of the development of day care. 'Meals-on-Wheels' may be required when the patient does not attend, and help from the Ministry of Social Security is often needed. Local-authority psychiatric social workers, mental welfare officers and health visitors are often able to help when patients fail to attend. Voluntary workers who have helped the patient in the past may continue to show interest which extends to a general interest in the day hospital. In a variety of ways, day care has widened the horizons of the hospital staff, introducing them to community organizations of which they had no knowledge. Community workers in turn have gained more insight into hospital activities and found new ways of solving their problems.

Unfortunately, it has not yet been possible to involve the family doctor in the day hospital and its associated services. Some general practitioners are employed as clinical assistants in the hospital, a few attend clinical meetings and lectures and one or two pay informal visits to the day unit. Simple forms are used in the day hospital to inform the family doctor and relatives of any changes, however slight, in treatment and care. These are completed by either a doctor or nurse, depending on the information being supplied. These small attempts on both sides help, but do not lead to true involvement. This problem will be discussed further in a later chapter.

It is difficult to assess the effectiveness of the day hospital in the same way as it is difficult to assess the usefulness of any type of community care. This question has been discussed in the previous chapter. A rough estimate of how many patients have been kept out of hospital and how many have been discharged since day care became available is possible. These figures do not measure patient well-being, community tolerance or impact on the family and tend to be a little inaccurate because they depend on the subjective judgements of medical and nursing staff.

Between December 1963 and March 1967, it is believed that 117 admissions were prevented and 137 discharges made possible. Some relatives have complained of the strain, even with full day hospital support, but the majority of interested and vocal relatives appear to be satisfied with the help provided. The provision of day care has also meant that many more patients and families have been helped than would have been possible if only in-patient care were available. This in itself is a major argument in favour of this type of service, but perhaps the best reason for day care is that patients prefer it to hospitalization.

THE FUTURE

Experience at Severalls and many other centres including Oxford and Worthing has shown that day hospitals can play an important part in keeping old people out of hospital. How effective they are in successfully supporting patients in the community, to the advantage of patient, relative and neighbour, requires further investigation. There is an obvious need for an extensive inquiry into this subject. If impressions are correct and day care is effective, certain modifications and developments are necessary. At present the hospital service is expected to provide day hospitals, while local authorities and voluntary organizations run day and occupational centres. Day hospitals for the elderly are often duplicated, one being provided for geriatric patients and another for psychogeriatric cases. An old person may require only day centre support. Later an illness may develop that could be treated in a day hospital, which means either transfer to a day hospital or – more likely – admission to hospital. A patient may attend a geriatric day unit, develop psychiatric symptoms and again be transferred or admitted. If comprehensive day centres were available, providing all facets of care, these problems would not arise. Old people attending this type of unit would be cared for regardless of the varying picture they may present from day to day. Day centre care would be improved because of the presence of skilled personnel, and day hospital patients would receive more overall care and benefit from an increased variety of occupation and entertainment. The only serious obstacle to such a scheme would be official inelasticity. It should be possible for local authority, voluntary organization and hospital board to arrive at some mutually satisfactory arrangement by which such centres could be accommodated, staffed and financed. Each organization would save money, economize in staff, and yet produce a better service for the patient.

Today, in spite of the great increase in the number of day hospitals and centres, day care is available only in limited areas of the country. There is an urgent need for a day unit or units in every centre of population. Sparsely populated areas present special problems. In these areas a small unit could cater for a large area. Experience at Severalls suggests that patients can come from a twenty-five mile radius with little discomfort or adverse effect on health. Staffing may be difficult, but country districts are often well supplied with voluntary workers. Village general practitioners may be persuaded to help, and if they do, will soon be encouraged to continue when they discover that the demands of their elderly patients are being met more satis-factorily without frequent home visits.

It has previously been claimed that day hospitals are more effective and cheaper to run if they are part of a hospi-tal. It would be possible to retain this advantage if compre-hensive units were located in hospital grounds. In rural areas the day unit could be associated with the local cottage hos-pital. Each area would develop a service depending on its needs and facilities.

Developments in the care of old people indicate that day care will become more widely used whatever final pattern evolves. To be successful, it must not operate in isolation but be an integral part of an overall service including in-patient and community care facilities. General practitioners need to be involved in the service to a greater degree than has been possible so far at Severalls. The staff of the day unit must be sufficiently interested to want it to develop and succeed. Active concern for patients must be experi-enced by all grades of staff. When a patient fails to attend, for example, it should be an automatic response from the staff to find out what has happened and act accordingly.

At Severalls it has been possible to foster this interest and concern by involving staff in specific projects, holding frequent informal meetings and by individual discussion and explanation. As the service grew, practical evidence of usefulness became available and interest spread from those involved to other workers in both hospital and com-munity. The well recognized but relatively little used tech-niques of administration that produce good communication, feelings of individual responsibility and identification with a project have played an important part in the success of day care at Severalls.

In the Service of Old Age

References

Cosin, L. Z., 'Organization of a Day Hospital for Psychotic Patients in a Geriatric Unit', *Proceedings of the Royal Society of Medicine*, May 1956, p. 237.

Farndale, J., *The Day Hospital Movement in Great Britain*, Pergamon Press, 1961.

Haider, I., 'A New Day Hospital Service', *British Journal of Psychiatry*, February 1967, pp. 173–4.

7 | The Emergency Service

The organization at Severalls has considerably reduced the number of unplanned admissions, but some still occur. In the early days of the unit, too many old people were admitted as emergencies. Some were emergencies in truth, but in many cases it appeared after they were in hospital that urgent admission could have been prevented. Conditions leading to a request for an admission as an emergency ranged from severely disturbed behaviour to mild nocturnal confusion associated with ill-advised night sedation with barbiturates. Often a breakdown of domestic arrangements was the real reason for requesting admission. A little personal mismanagement, lack of money and no support from the appropriate community services had led to a poorly stocked larder, no coal and a general structural deterioration of the home. If the old person was discovered in this condition, particularly in the evening or at night, emergency admission to somewhere was usually the only solution considered. Evidence of memory defect, however slight, or abnormal emotional behaviour usually meant a referral to the psychiatric hospital.

Evenings, nights and week-ends had the highest incidence of requests for emergency admission. These are times when it is difficult to mobilize community services and it was considered that admission could often have been prevented if appropriate personnel had been available to deal with the situation in the home. These cases led to the development of a domiciliary emergency service at Severalls.

THE DEVELOPMENT OF THE EMERGENCY SERVICE

In 1961, nurses at Severalls became actively involved in community care, visiting selected patients in their homes. This was done in cooperation with local-authority workers and was a variant of a scheme operating in Croydon (May and Moore, 1963). Social workers employed by the hospital also started to play a more active part in community investigation and support.

When the unit was reorganized in 1963 and a planned admission procedure introduced, the formation of a team to deal with emergencies was considered. The increased use of day care at this time made it easier to support patients referred as emergencies, provided the immediate situation could be dealt with in the home. The extension of day care to patients who would previously have been admitted also made it necessary to devise some system for dealing with patients who failed to attend the day hospital or became suddenly disturbed at home. Local-authority mental welfare officers were sometimes able to help with these cases, but pressure of work often precluded an immediate visit and delay sometimes led to admission.

It was suggested that a team should be formed consisting of a doctor, one or two nurses and a social worker. The team would be available to go out at any time, the actual members being selected on each occasion from a list of those who had volunteered and were available. They would carry equipment and supplies to cope with both clinical and social problems, and be willing to do whatever was necessary in the home, regardless of its nature.

The equipment to be carried (see list on pp. 101–102) included medical and surgical supplies, cleaning materials, food, fuel and tools for doing simple repairs. If possible an ambulance would be used as transport in case admission was necessary. One nurse in the team would be available to act as a night sitter if one was needed. It was suggested that the service should be limited to an area within a twenty-mile radius of Colchester. To cover the whole catchment area would have been impracticable because of the long journeys this would involve.

Unfortunately, prolonged negotiations took place between the hospital, the Regional Hospital Board and the local authority before it was possible to start the project as originally planned. In spite of this, a less ambitious service did start in 1964. When an emergency occurred a social worker, a doctor with a social worker or nurse, a social worker and a nurse, or two nurses would go to the home, using their own transport. They would deal with the problem when possible without admitting the patient. No night sitters were available, but many admissions were prevented in this way. The service was used only with the approval of the patient's general practitioner and all cases were seen and examined by a unit doctor either in the home or in the day hospital. Towards the end of 1965 the full service came into operation, agreement having been reached with the local authority and the Regional Hospital Board. The provision of night sitters still remained a problem. The normal night sitter service is provided by local authorities, who maintain a panel of people willing to do this type of work when required. Payment is on an hourly basis. The majority of night sitters are women with little formal nursing experience. They are not expected to provide nursing care, their function being to furnish family-type support and company at night for patients being nursed at home. Their help is usually sought for patients who are physically ill or dying and they tend to be unfamiliar with psychiatric syndromes. It is usually possible to obtain one if required, but their lack of training and experience limits their use. Difficulties do occur if one is wanted in an emergency and it is usually impossible to make the necessary arrangements at night or at the week-end. Because of these difficulties it was thought advisable to make arrangements with emergency team members to act as night sitters when necessary: the idea being that they would care for the patient at night until a local authority-employed sitter could be obtained or the patient no longer required the service.

Little difficulty was experienced obtaining volunteers even when it was explained that working as a night sitter was independent of hospital duties and would not entitle them to time off during the day. The volunteers were available but administrative difficulties remained. Long discussions took place involving the Regional Hospital Board, Group Treasurer's Department and the local authority. Problems dealt with included how payments should be made, who should pay, insurance cover and legal responsibility. These were all proper things to discuss, but the resulting delay tended to produce staff despondency and waning interest. It was to the credit of all concerned that a great deal of trouble was taken with these problems and a solution finally produced. The final arrangement was that the doctor responsible for the emergency service would inform the hospital treasurer's department and the local medical officer of health when a nurse or other hospital employee was used as a night sitter, giving details of hours spent in the patient's home. The hospital would then pay the staff member for the hours worked and recoup the money from the local authority. Payment by the local authority was considered necessary because of the administrative and financial structure of the health service.

It was now possible to operate the full service and supply a range of emergency help, from a visit by a social worker or nurse to the full team complete with potential night sitter.

STAFF INTEREST, USE AND EFFECT

The unit medical, nursing, social work and secretarial staff became interested in the project during the early planning stages. Their interest soon spread to staff in other units and departments. A panel of volunteers who were willing to act as team members when required soon included the unit's medical staff, two social workers, assistant matron and assistant chief male nurse. Eight male and eleven female nurses volunteered, together with one of the hospital pharmacists and a porter. The nurses included sisters, charge nurses, staff nurses, student and assistant nurses. Three male nurses, three female nurses, the hospital pharmacist and the porter agreed to act as night sitters when necessary. Local-authority mental health workers showed considerable interest and agreed to help the team at any time they were free of other duties and available. One mental welfare officer asked to be informed whenever the team was used so that he could assist as often as possible.

From January 1964 to August 1966, 170 emergency visits were made to 109 patients (Figure 5). On four occasions

Reason for referral	Number of referrals	Result of visit		
		Day Hospital care	Community care with Day Hospital attendance	Admitted to Hospital
Disturbed behaviour	55	17	20	18
Patients failing to care for themselves	103	48	40	15
Physical illness in Day Patients	12	3	5	4
Totals	170	68	65	37

Figure 5. Cases dealt with by the Emergency Service between January 1964 and August 1966

the full team was used, night sitters being required for one, two or three nights. The other cases were dealt with by a social worker or some other variant of the smaller team. Sixty-eight patients needed only to be brought to the day hospital and sixty-five required day care and help in the home. The latter included domestic cleaning, stocking the larder, minor repairs or laying a fire for the evening before the patient came to the day hospital. Thirty-seven patients were admitted. Fifty-five cases were referred because of disturbed behaviour and 103 because they were neglecting themselves. Twelve day patients who had developed physical illnesses are included in the total cases dealt with.

The usefulness of the emergency service is as difficult to assess as any other community treatment and supportive service. The difficulties have already been discussed in relation to community care and the day hospital. From the statistics available, seventy-two admissions were prevented between January 1964 and August 1966, making a yearly average of twenty-seven. During the same period the number of in-patients was reduced by ninety-nine. From these figures it would appear that the emergency service played a significant part in reducing the in-patient load and making community care work. However, even at this simple level of measurement it is difficult to assess the part played by any one facet of the service in producing overall effects. For example, without a day hospital the results of using the emergency service would have been very different, since the majority of cases dealt with were considered to require day care.

ILLUSTRATIVE CASES

Case 1

A widow of 82 was referred by her general practitioner for compulsory emergency admission. Having neglected herself and her small bungalow for some months, she was now causing concern by wandering abroad at night, not eating, and appearing in the road half dressed. She had refused treatment and would not go to hospital.

The general practitioner agreed to a visit by the emergency team. This was carried out by a unit social worker and nurse in the social worker's car. They were able to persuade the old lady to come to the day hospital.

On examination she was found to be depressed, with little evidence of dementia. Treatment as a day patient, with food, vitamins and anti-depressants produced a rapid improvement. The home help organization dealt with the bungalow. During the first two weeks of treatment she failed to attend on two occasions, but the day hospital sister and social worker visited her each time and were able to persuade her to come back to the day unit. She attended daily for six weeks by which time she had improved sufficiently to manage at home and only visited the day hospital one day each week.

Case 2

A widower of 88 was referred by his general practitioner one Sunday afternoon. Over a period of two to three weeks he had become progressively more unsteady on his feet. He had fallen out of bed on the two previous nights, and was now unable to stand. He lived alone, and had no one to look after him except a neighbour who could only look in occasionally.

With the approval of the general practitioner, he was visited by the team. On this occasion a local-authority ambulance was used, the team consisting of a doctor, social worker, male assistant matron, male charge nurse and male student nurse. An ambulance was used because it was considered admission might be necessary.

When the team arrived at the cottage the patient was in bed. He was drowsy, but there was no evidence of specific disease. There was no food in the house and the cooking stove had not been used for some time. Apparently he had been taking tranquillizers prescribed by his doctor.

While the nurses washed the patient and made the bed, other members of the team tidied the home, prepared some food and obtained what information they could from the neighbour. A nurse was left with the patient for the night, both coming into the day hospital by ambulance the next day.

Regular meals, physiotherapy and no tranquillizers effected a rapid recovery, but for the next two nights it was thought advisable to have someone stay with him. On one night a female student nurse acted as night sitter and on the other a hospital pharmacist took on this role. No further night supervision was considered necessary, but the patient continued to attend the day hospital.

Case 3

A domiciliary visit was requested to a widow of 67 with a view to compulsory admission. Following the death of her husband a year previously, she had lived alone. During this period she had become progressively more depressed and less able to manage. On the day of the referral she had removed some furniture from her home to the garden, burned some of her clothes and told her doctor that people were trying to get her out of the house.

Her general practitioner agreed to a visit bb the emergency team. A preliminary visit was made by a unit social worker and nurse. They were able to persuade the patient to come to the day hospital. Before bringing her in they replaced the furniture and tidied the house, helped by the patient. A son was visited who found someone to stay with his mother in the home at night.

Treatment for her depression in the day hospital produced

a satisfactory recovery and she was soon able to return to a normal life.

Some may consider that the work done by the emergency team should be the responsibility of the local authority. This may be true, but few authorities could provide this type of service. The pattern of development of psychiatric hospitals is for their staff to become more involved in community work. In this way hospital staff gain a greater understanding of patients and their families, cooperation with other community workers is increased and something approaching continuity of care is possible. The emergency service has been a further extension of this movement. It has augmented existing community services without operating in competition with them, and community workers have welcomed the help offered. The service has operated successfully only because there were other forms of support available after the emergency was over.

There is another advantage in the hospital running this kind of service. In hospital a variety of staff with diverse skills are easily available. It would be difficult for any local authority to have available such personnel who could be mobilized quickly and few authorities have skilled nurses trained both in general and psychiatric nursing.

The original idea of a full team using an ambulance has been modified. Experience has shown that the majority of cases can be dealt with by one or two team members, using their own transport. If they are unable to cope, the full team can always be mobilized and sent to their assistance.

An important factor in the efficient working of the service has been the willingness of team members to do any job that may be necessary to maintain the patient in the community. These have included moving furniture, lighting fires, preparing food, carrying out minor repairs and collecting food from the local shops. The formation of the emergency team has again illustrated how staff attitudes are changed when they are involved in an interesting project and allowed to use their initiative. Doctors, nurses, social workers and other staff have ceased to be concerned with their specific roles and done jobs normally considered outside their sphere and beneath their dignity.

All the staff involved in the project have developed a greater respect for each other, so disproving the belief that rigid observation of role is necessary for the maintenance of professional status. The service has also demonstrated how the present structure of the Health Service need not be a block to developing programmes that cut across administrative dividing lines.

Many branches of medicine are now becoming concerned with preventing admissions and dealing with patients in their own home. A very successful paediatric home-nursing service has been in operation in Paddington for the past ten years (Bergman, Shrand and Oppé, 1965). The emergency service at Severalls deals only with old people with presumed psychiatric illness. There does not appear to be any legitimate reason why the same team or a similar one could not deal with other types of emergency involving the elderly. Experience in general psychiatry would also indicate a need for such a service to deal with younger psychiatric patients who suddenly become disturbed or are referred for emergency admission because of social and domestic crises.

References

Bergman, A. B., Shrand, H., and Oppé, T. E., 'A Paediatric Home Care Programme in London – Ten Years' Experience', *Paediatrics*, September 1965.

May, A. R., and Moore, S., 'The Mental Nurse in the Community', *Lancet*, 26 January 1963.

LIST OF EQUIPMENT CARRIED BY EMERGENCY TEAM

Medical and Nursing

1 medicine box
Elastoplast
2 zinc-oxide viscopaste bandages
6 bandages at 2″ gauze
4 bandages at 3″ crêpe
1 packet cotton wool
1 packet gauze
assorted catheters –
        size 10 upwards
tube and funnel with glass
        connexion
2 receivers
2 small bowls
2 galley pots
1 syringe 2 cc.
1 syringe 5 cc.
1 syringe 10 cc.
12 needles
1 pair surgical gloves
6 emergency suture packs
1 pair dissecting forceps
1 pair artery forceps
1 pair scissors

1 bottle methylated spirit
1 bottle olive oil
1 bottle soluble insulin
1 jar glucose
intravenous glucose –
        2 ampoules
adrenaline 1: 1,000–
        6 ampoules
morphia grains $\frac{1}{4}$ – 6 ampoules
mersalyl – 6 ampoules
aminophylline 10 ml. –
        5 ampoules
digoxin 0.25 mg. – 25 tablets
Crystamycin – 5 ampoules
oxy-tetracycline – 20 tablets
dichloralphenazone (Welldorm)
        – 20 tablets
promethazine (Phenergen)
        25 mg. – 20 tablets
promazine (Sparine) 50 mg. –
        20 tablets
1 tube silicone cream
distilled water – 5 ampoules

Domestic

1 gallon paraffin
1 pair rubber boots
2 packets fire lighters
1 bag coal
1 broom
1 Imp soot dispeller
1 powdered scourer
2 tablets soap
3 electric light bulbs
1 portable Botogaz stove
6 boxes matches
1 dozen candles
fuse wire

1 bottle of liquid detergent
1 pail
1 brush and dustpan
3 floor cloths
3 dusters
1 bottle of disinfectant
2 pillows
4 sheets
2 towels
2 face cloths
1 dozen incontinence sheets
1 box tissues
1 comb

In the Service of Old Age

Domestic (continued)

needle and thread
1 ball white tape
1 sickle
1 spade
1 roll wide Sellotape
1 ball of string
6 sheets brown paper
2 rolls toilet paper
1 small hammer
½ lb. assorted nails

1 screwdriver
3 small tins of soup
tea and sugar
10s. 0d. worth assorted coins
1 dozen plastic bags 10″ × 8″
1 torch
4 cotton cellular bankets
3 small tins of Ideal milk
1 tin opener

8 | The In-Patient Service

In spite of emphasis being placed on supporting old people outside hospital a number still need to be admitted and some have to remain there until they die. There is always a danger of concentrating interest and resources on the patient who can be maintained in the community or discharged from hospital at the expense of those who remain as in-patients. The terms 'long-stay', 'chronics', 'unrecoverables', often convey an affect of abandonment and neglect. A paper in the *Lancet* (Little, 1963) on the future of psychiatric hospitals appeared to suggest that this attitude should be perpetuated. It was claimed that treatable patients should be dealt with in general hospital units while so-called 'unrecoverables' would go to the mental hospital now staffed by part-time general practitioners and assistant nurses. Fortunately, a large body of psychiatrists, geriatricians and nurses does not agree with this approach to patients who may appear to be beyond help.

The risk of long-stay patients being treated as second- or third-rate citizens is always present. An attempt is being made in the majority of psychiatric hospitals, including Severalls, to combat this danger. The degree of success has varied from hospital to hospital and from time to time. The Severalls psychogeriatric in-patient unit has had the same varied success but the goal has always been the equal treatment of all patients. Treatment and rehabilitation have been used to prepare patients for return to the community and to improve the lives of those who have to remain in hospital indefinitely.

It may be considered unrealistic to talk of rehabilitating

elderly psychiatric patients, particularly when they are suffering from the effects of chronic brain damage. Unfortunately, rehabilitation is too often looked upon as simply improving the work-potential of younger patients so they can be returned to useful employment after discharge. Some consider rehabilitation to be making the patient more acceptable to society. Thus emphasis is too often placed on making the patient fit in and be useful to the community. These may be reasonable, if rather limited, aims but disregard the patient as an individual. One meaning of the word rehabilitate is 'give back dignity' and this is what a rehabilitation programme should be about. Old people with mental illness have often lost their dignity. Memory defect, incontinence, the reactions of relatives and the effects of admission to hospital, all may have worked together to destroy the patient's self-respect. Every geriatric and psychogeriatric unit needs a rehabilitation programme designed to restore self-respect as well as prepare patients for life outside hospital. The patient who will never leave is in the greatest need. Those who are discharged from hospital may regain their dignity by becoming independent again. Those who remain cannot improve unless help is provided.

The efficiency of an in-patient service like any other service depends upon it not becoming overloaded. Overloading can be prevented by an effective community care programme and the careful screening of admissions. An admission procedure and a planned use of in-patient facilities have been in operation at Severalls since 1961, some modifications occurring in 1963.

ADMISSION PROCEDURE

As emphasized before, the admission of an old person to hospital should always be looked upon as a serious step and never advised without careful consideration of the total situation which has led to the request for in-patient care. Patients should never be admitted because of academic interest, to allay a doctor's anxiety or as a quick solution to a difficult social problem. Legitimate reasons for admission can be considered under three headings:

(i) The need for treatment that is not possible on a domiciliary out-patient or day-patient basis.

(ii) The impossibility of containing the patient in the community because of behaviour or inadequacies in community care.

(iii) The need to give relatives and friends a respite and rest in order for them to continue care after the patient has been in hospital for a limited period.

The help given to relatives and friends can range from a short admission while they take a holiday, to a regular month-in/month-out routine, the latter being a variation of a concept originally described by De Largy (1957). In this way the care of the patient is shared between the hospital and the family, the patient does not feel rejected, and always has something to look forward to and is not cut off from the community. The family are better able to cope and usually become more tolerant, and the hospital is able to provide help for a larger number of patients and their families.

Figure 6 (p. 106) illustrates the service provided by the unit and shows the fluid nature of the support that may be provided. Support must vary, depending on the immediate needs of patient and family.

To operate a service on these principles, it is important for all admissions to be planned. Patients and relatives or friends must be seen before admission, in order to decide upon a mutually acceptable plan. This can be done by a doctor or social worker, depending on the condition of the patient, the urgency of the situation and the availability of

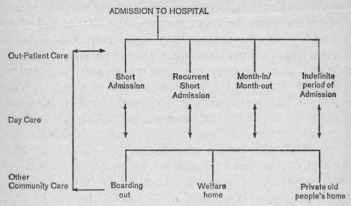

Figure 6. Types of in-patient care offered by the psychogeriatric unit

staff. Whenever possible a combined assessment is carried out. Emergencies and urgent requests for admission can sometimes present difficulties, but, provided staff orientation and interest are satisfactory, it is usually possible to use the method described. The development of the emergency service has played an important part in solving these problems.

It was possible to develop a special relationship with the local authority Welfare Department regarding transfer of patients from their old people's homes to the unit. Soon after the unit was set up, difficulties occurred with transfers from these homes which threatened good relations between Welfare Department and hospital. Few transfers occurred from hospital to welfare home. Contact with the Welfare Department was establishd through a variety of informal meetings with the county welfare officer and members of his staff. A system was devised that made transfer rapid and easy, with advantage to patient, hospital and welfare home. If a resident of a welfare home became disturbed or for other reasons required transfer to the unit, it was agreed that his place in the home would be kept for a period of six weeks in the first place, with the possibility of extension if necessary. In order that scarce accommodation should be fully utilized, arrangements were also made for a patient from the unit to take the vacant welfare-home place. This was done on a holiday basis and only with the full agreement of the patient, who was usually awaiting a place in a welfare home or accommodation under the boarding-out scheme. If the patient from the welfare home recovered sufficiently to return, the patient filling the place returned to the unit. If recovery did not occur, the patient from the unit still returned unless it happened that he was due for transfer to a welfare home or had settled in the home to such a degree that return to hospital might be damaging to his well-being.

This arrangement had a number of advantages. Patients from welfare homes can be admitted quickly regardless of the unit bed state. Their place in the home is kept open, always making return possible unless their condition is such that improvement is highly unlikely. Patients from the unit can have a temporary change of environment and their ability to cope when away from the hospital can be measured under controlled conditions. This helps assessment of their chances of successful settling outside hospital before they are finally boarded out or discharged to welfare or private old people's homes. Trading in human bodies, typified by the system of swapping patients between hospitals or hospital and welfare home, does not occur. The patient from the unit goes willingly, knowing that he will either return to the hospital after a limited period, or remain permanently in the welfare home if there is mutual agreement. The use of this system and regular meetings that developed between hospital and Welfare Department staff appear to have created a good relationship between the two services and increased the number of patients transferred from hospital to welfare accommodation.

THE IN-PATIENT UNIT

The in-patient unit consists of two male, four female and two mixed ground-floor wards, catering for 107 men and 170 women and dealing with a catchment area population of 750,000. The mixed wards either have male patients in the dormitory portion and female in the smaller side wards, or women in the dormitory and men in the side wards. One mixed ward is used for intensive rehabilitation of long-stay patients being prepared for discharge under the unit's boarding-out scheme or to relatives or to Welfare Department accommodation. Two wards have double rooms set aside for the admission of married couples. When a married couple both need admission to hospital or welfare home, it is bizarrely inhuman to separate them, and when one member of a couple with close emotional ties requires admission, it should be possible to admit them together. The trauma of separation is prevented, misery reduced, and often care in hospital is made easier because of the help provided by the relatively fit partner.

Mixed wards were introduced because it was considered unnatural, artificial and anti-therapeutic to segregate the sexes. All wards were not mixed because of administrative and nursing difficulties. Experience has shown the need for some single-sex wards. A few patients and staff object to mixed wards, feel threatened by the presence of the opposite sex or behave in a manner unacceptable in mixed company. The ratio of mixed to unmixed wards in the unit is possibly wrong and should be reversed, leaving only two single-sex wards.

The advantages of mixing patients have been obvious; their behaviour has improved, they have taken more interest in their appearance and a livelier atmosphere has been created. This has confirmed the findings of staff in the few psychiatric hospitals and general hospital psychiatric units in Britain and the U.S.A. where younger patients of both sexes are treated in the same wards. Most of the staff who first looked upon this innovation with doubts and fears soon realized the advantages and after a time forgot there was anything unusual about men and women living in the same ward.

When the unit was opened the wards were organized into a pattern of progressive care. Nursing care and facilities were concentrated in the admission wards, and when patients improved they were transferred to other wards with progressively decreasing nursing care and increasing independence on the part of the patients. There are certain advantages to this system, but there are also some obvious disadvantages. Old people, on the whole, react badly to change and often have difficulty in developing new relationships and learning new geography. Some patients improve following admission, only to relapse when transferred to another ward. Because of these serious problems the system was changed. Patients were admitted to wards considered appropriate for their needs and movement from ward to ward was reduced to a minimum, occurring only for adequate reasons. Patients were moved because of their needs, not because of system or administrative convenience.

WARD LAYOUT AND FURNISHINGS

All wards in the unit are on the ground floor and have easy access to gardens – an arrangement possible in many hospitals. This results in more freedom for patients, encourages them to spend time in the gardens and visit other parts of the hospital and makes visiting easier for elderly relatives and friends.

Each ward has separate dining- and sitting-rooms, and where possible, extra space is provided for entertainment and industrial therapy. Where this is not practicable these activities are carried out in sitting or dining-rooms. It is the policy of the hospital to encourage patients to work and to be entertained outside the ward but some old people have physical disabilities that make movement about the hospital difficult, hence the need for some provision in the ward for these activities.

Because privacy is usually valued by patients, dormitories are divided into four-bed areas by using specially designed wardrobe/dressing-table units. These units provide adequate space for clothes and personal possessions and somewhere for a friendly ornament or photograph which can improve patient morale and reduce feelings of isolation and abandonment. Side rooms are also used to provide privacy and not as punishment cells for the so-called difficult patients.

The standard hospital bed was originally designed to facilitate the nursing of patients confined to bed because most physically ill patients were treated in bed and psychiatric patients were not considered. The average height of a standard hospital bed is 28 inches compared to 17 inches for a modern divan bed. Mobile old people find them inconvenient and sometimes frightening and their use leads to falls unless this is prevented by turning them into cages with cot sides. Incontinence is encouraged, since a trip to the lavatory becomes a dangerous adventure. Low beds do not have these disadvantages and are used in most wards in the unit, some standard beds being retained for patients requiring temporary confinement to bed. In this way nurses' backs are preserved without all patients being penalized.

Even in an active unit, many patients spend long periods in chairs. The chairs provided cater for the needs of elderly patients, being high enough to facilitate sitting and rising, with well-shaped high backs that fully support the head and trunk. There has been much discussion about the use of geriatric chairs with fixed trays. These can be used as a form of restraint to prevent patients wandering, or as a prison for a 'difficult' patient, but used properly, they can fulfil a useful function. Many long-stay patients have been confined to bed for years, and their mobilization can take time and sometimes is not fully successful. These chairs can then play a part in progressive mobilization and make life a little easier for those who never become fully ambulant. They are used for limited periods only, the patients spending part of the day doing walking exercises, part in other activities and part resting on their beds. It is important to keep old people active, but this should not mean preventing them from having a nap in the afternoon.

Lavatory, washing and bathing facilities are made easily available to all patients, and nurses are encouraged to spend time teaching patients the ward geography. Patient mobility can be increased by providing wall bars that afford physical and moral support for the anxious and infirm. These have not yet been fitted in the wards, but are part of the programme for future developments.

TREATMENT

In every age some people have realized that the sick require more than the specific remedy if they are to be helped. They have known that treatment consists of dealing with the patient as a whole, his environment and his relationships with others. This approach is time-consuming and involves the therapist in problems outside the narrow confines of medicine, which is possibly one reason why treatment still tends to be looked upon as consisting of pills, the use of standard nursing procedures, physiotherapy, surgery, electroplexy and circumscribed psychotherapy. Good treatment for the mentally-ill is much more than this and the therapist must concern himself with the patient's environment as well as the patient's symptoms. Good treatment includes: unrestricted visiting; suitable ward furnishing and décor; the provision of newspapers, magazines and books; conversation; asking not telling; allowing for any idiosyncrasies; providing money for patients to spend; the provision of spectacles, hearing aids, dentures; and respect for the individual. When this broader concept of treatment is accepted institutional neurosis becomes rare, patients recover more quickly and are much less likely to suffer because they came into hospital.

An attempt has been made at Severalls to provide a setting in which patients are treated like adults and not like recalcitrant children. Visiting is unrestricted, patients are encouraged to keep their own possessions, and furniture is provided to make this possible. Pride in appearance is engendered by allowing patients to buy their own clothes or select what they want to wear if hospital clothing is provided. Mirrors are plentiful and a beauty salon is located in the hospital.

Conversation, entertainment and occupation are considered more important than traditional nursing techniques. Most nurses enjoy nursing, which unfortunately can lead to patients being kept in bed, to hand feeding, bathing by nurses, obsessional interest in bowel activity, over-protection and the final conversion of an adult into a helpless baby. The more dedicated and industrious the nurse, the greater the danger. A constant programme of re-education carried out in a sympathetic, supportive manner is necessary and nurses have to be shown the practical advantages and humanity of allowing patients to care for themselves, with help, but with the minimum of interference and impatience.

The elderly, like most people, appear to benefit from occupation. Most psychiatric hospitals provide three types:

industrial therapy, traditional occupational therapy and hospital work. Industrial therapy should be meaningful, produce a saleable end product and result in financial reward. Traditional occupational therapy tends to be concerned with crafts and provides satisfaction in doing and creating something. Hospital work, which can range from domestic duties in the ward to employment in the laundry, is a relic of the past and the last example of slavery in this country. As far as possible, patients in the unit are allowed to choose what they want to do, since preparation for earning a living outside hospital is not usually the object of treatment. Something to occupy part of the day which incites interest, gives satisfaction and increases social contact is the goal. Therapy in the household management unit is a partial exception. Here, patients are re-educated in household duties, including meal planning, cooking and washing. Treatment is designed to prepare patients for returning home, but some who may never leave hospital attend as part of a programme to re-establish self-respect.

An important provision for all old people, however demented they appear, is conversation. Possibly much of the success claimed for individual and group psychotherapy in psychogeriatric practice is due to the opportunity provided for conversation. Nurses and doctors in the unit are expected to spend as much time as possible talking to patients. This is considered more valuable than many nursing rituals and the unrewarding, and usually pointless, routine yearly physical examination, no longer statutory but still carried out obsessionally in some institutions.

Urinary and faecal incontinence can be a major problem in any geriatric unit. There is no overall answer since the aetiology is varied. Dementia plays a part, but immobility, local causes – particularly cystitis and constipation – psychotic and neurotic reactions, misuse of sedatives and tranquillizers and over-protection are all likely to contribute in producing this unpleasant and demoralizing condition. Physiotherapy, low beds, easy access to toilets, treatment of underlying psychiatric and physical disease, activity and reawakening of interests, increased social contacts and habit training, can usually produce dramatic improvements. One ward in the unit had a seventy per cent incidence of incontinence reduced to ten per cent when the staff paid attention to these factors. The combination of habit training and use of anti-cholinergic drugs usually reduces the frequency of incontinence even in the most resistant cases.

Simple refinements to a ward can play an important part in improving the quality of patients' lives but staff are often so preoccupied with nursing procedures, physical treatments and the keeping of records that they forget or ignore anything else.

The provision of papers, books and magazines; a mobile shop; properly served food; milk, sugar and butter on the table; bowls of flowers; pictures; curtains on the window; a television and radio that can be operated by patients; free access to the ward kitchen; a notice board with a clear calendar and information about the hospital and its activities: all are essentials. Nurses working in the unit are encouraged to institute changes in the ward layout, activity and routine. In this way, steady improvement in patient care continues and staff interest is maintained.

The ward is not the only place of activity. Every patient who is able to leave the ward is encouraged to go to the occupational therapy or industrial therapy departments, the hospital shop, beauty salon, household management unit, and any other place of occupation or entertainment inside or outside the hospital precinct. Walks in the grounds or outside the hospital are organized, even with staff shortages. Friends and relatives are usually willing to help and many patients go unaccompanied, sometimes taking less able friends with them. The traditional institutional practice of taking large numbers of patients for walks in 'crocodiles' guarded by bored nurses is strongly discouraged, since it turns what should be a pleasant social occasion into a prison activity.

The usual range of more conventional treatments are provided, including the use of various drugs for psychiatric and physical illness, electro-convulsive therapy, psychotherapy, physiotherapy and surgery. Experience has shown that their efficacy is greatly enhanced when attention is paid to atmosphere and to the encouragement of social activity, occupation and self-respect.

RELATIVES AND FRIENDS

The importance of relatives and friends in the social and clinical assessment of the patient and the need to interest and involve them in the therapeutic situation will be discussed in Chapter 10. They are mentioned here because this important subject warrants some repetition. Relatives and friends may be the only link patients have with the outside world and the patients' resettlement in the community usually depends on their interest, involvement and goodwill. In spite of this, some doctors and nurses treat them like the enemy, avoiding interviews and dismissing queries with vague, uninterested answers. They need to be made welcome in the hospital, their interest should be encouraged and cooperation developed.

Unrestricted visiting, invitation to the social activities in the hospital, relatives' conferences, individual and group meetings and staff education have helped to improve relationships with relatives and friends at Severalls.

Many hospitals do not allow visiting by children. This is tragically foolish – the perpetuation of rigid Victorian Poor Law attitudes. Children come to no harm, while patients almost always benefit. When children enter a ward, the whole atmosphere changes, dulled eyes brighten, smiles displace apathy, and long silences are ended. Children have always been welcome in the unit and they have never caused any trouble, or been upset by the experience, while the patients have obviously enjoyed their company.

Relatives are often elderly, lonely and sometimes in need of help. The unit staff are encouraged to interest themselves in relatives' welfare. As a result, many relatives and friends have come under treatment themselves; some have become day patients, while others have been assisted by mobilizing community services. It is believed that this has prevented a number of admissions and made possible the discharge of patients who would otherwise have remained in hospital because of unsatisfactory home conditions.

STAFFING, GROUP ACTIVITY AND STAFF INVOLVEMENT

The unit system has been described in Chapter 4. The psychogeriatric unit is under the control of a consultant psychiatrist, helped by a medical assistant and two or three junior doctors, an assistant matron, assistant chief male nurse, two social workers and two medical secretaries. The wards have the normal staff structure and, like every other psychiatric hospital, are under-staffed. What would be considered realistic, adequate staffing is difficult to judge, since it would appear to be an unalterable law that, whatever the number, staffing is always considered insufficient. Inadequate staffing is often used as an excuse for failing to improve services. It is not a valid reason. The quality of any psychiatric service, like any human activity, depends on the motivation, interest and attitudes of the personnel involved. Numbers help, but are not all-important. Motivation that is in tune with the project, interest that is maintained, and satisfactory attitudes can lead to the development of an effective and progressive service in the face of most difficulties.

The care of the elderly is too often looked upon as uninteresting and unrewarding. It tends to be unpopular and staff are frequently poorly motivated, uninformed and resistant to change. One important advantage of a separate unit for the elderly in a psychiatric hospital is that staff who are interested and willing to learn can be specifically recruited. Staff who show interest can be transferred from other parts of the hospital, while new staff can be specially selected for work in the unit.

A number of well-recognized methods have been used at Severalls to educate and involve all grades of medical, nursing and ancillary staff. Symposia, lectures, seminars, clinical meetings, visits to other hospitals and the provision of books and journals are all used as part of a constant educational programme. Education along these formal and semi-formal lines is never enough. Interest, willingness to learn and feelings of personal involvement can come only from example, good communication and a system that depends upon committing staff groups to specific projects. Methods of creating staff interest and involvement have included frequent, regular ward and unit meetings, which are informal and free, similar meetings with community workers, the use of nurses for community work and the development of specific projects and services by individual wards and staff groups. The emergency service, the boarding-out scheme and mixed rehabilitation wards are examples of group projects involving nurses, social workers, ancillary staff and doctors.

Research, aside from its usefulness *per se*, can also help in creating better staff attitudes. Evidence accumulated since Elton Mayo pioneered the study of human relationships in organizations with his research at the Hawthorne Plant of the Western Electric Company near Chicago between 1927 and 1932 (Roethlisberger and Dickson, 1939; Revans, 1966) has shown that morale can be significantly improved when members of the staff feel that they are a subject of interest and concern and are encouraged to use their own initiative and intelligence.

Ideas for research put forward by any worker in the unit are carefully considered and encouraged, provided there is no danger to patients. The results of many investigations may not be of any great significance, but the actual work carried out usually benefits both staff and patients.

Ward and unit meetings are conducted to improve communication, educate, and provide a psychotherapeutic milieu. Individual discussion and counselling with staff complement these group activities. Each Saturday morning the assistant psychiatrist to the unit carries out a staff round. The object is to talk to as many individual staff members as possible about their problems, ideas and complaints. This kind of discussion is not limited to Saturday mornings but the weekly round ensures that a regular pattern of discussion develops.

Patients are sometimes kept in hospital longer than necessary, discharged without satisfactory after-care and even forgotten. This is particularly likely to happen when staff numbers are inadequate. With these problems in mind, daily staff meetings were started. These are attended by the unit doctors, senior nurses and social workers. Details of patients due for admission and the problems of rehabilitation and discharge are fully discussed. These meetings also offer another opportunity for education and general discussion of the unit's problems and staff anxieties. Every Thursday morning, all patients admitted for short or limited periods are reviewed. Progress is checked, discharge dates arranged and modification to the original plan made on admission is discussed and implemented. The result of these meetings is that patients are unlikely to be forgotten, after-care is not overlooked and varied ideas are obtained about any problem or patient.

This description of the in-patient service may be considered self-satisfied. There is no self-satisfaction in the unit. A recent survey of staff attitudes, carried out as part of a general nursing survey in the hospital, has demonstrated a number of failings in education, attitude and motivation. New attempts are now being made to remedy these failings. The survey has demonstrated the importance of frequent re-examination of any organization. In this way complacency is kept under control and the development of fixed ideas is prevented. Before the results of the survey were available, many faults were acknowledged and many problems remained unsolved. Some staff members continue to believe that demented patients do not have any appreciation of their surroundings, so that it does not matter how food is served or wards decorated and furnished. These views are held in spite of the same persons complaining that several demented patients are disturbed after visits by relatives and friends and upset if moved to another ward.

Older members of staff, used to a rigid, authoritarian régime, have found it difficult to adapt to increased freedom and informality. Having been used to ordering patients about, some find it difficult to use persuasion, and tend to continue in the old way or otherwise swing to an extreme *laissez-faire* attitude which usually means that patients do nothing, spending the day staring hopelessly into space.

There are still complains about 'difficult' patients. This sometimes means that a patient is behaving in an abnormal or disturbed manner, which is indeed one good reason for his being in hospital, where he can benefit from the special skills psychiatrists and psychiatric nurses should possess. Sometimes the 'difficult' patient is the well patient, intolerant of hospital routine and staff rigidity. In either case the situation should be understood and dealt with skilfully; it should not result in complaints or punishment by confinement in a side room or in the geriatric chair.

Some advantages of a separate psychogeriatric in-patient unit have been mentioned. The special problems of old people can be catered for and a programme of activity devised that combats institutionalism yet remains leisurely enough for this age group. A serious disadvantage is that the old are segregated from the young. An attempt has been made to remedy this fault by encouraging young patients to visit the unit and work on the wards. Young patients with personality disorders are often a great help, tend to be liked by the elderly and behave better than in other situations. Whenever possible, elderly patients go to activities outside the ward where they meet younger patients. Unrestricted visiting and allowing children in the ward have also helped to remedy the ill effects of segregation.

Some members of staff still do not like working on the psychogeriatric wards but the majority find the work interesting and rewarding. It is considered that experience in the psychogeriatric unit not only helps them to understand the problems of the elderly but also provides useful experience that can be utilized in any branch of psychiatry or nursing.

References

De Largy, J., 'Six weeks in; Six weeks out. A Geriatric Hospital Scheme for Rehabilitating the Aged and Relieving their Relatives', *Lancet*, 23 February 1957, pp. 418–19.

Little, J. Crawford, 'A Rational Plan for Integration of Psychiatric Services to an Urban Community', *Lancet*, 30 November 1963, pp. 1,159–60.

Revans, R. W., *Standards for Morale – Cause and Effect in Hospitalization*, Oxford University Press, 1966.

Roethlisberger, F. J., and Dickson, W. J., *Management and the Worker*, Oxford University Press, 1939.

9 | Boarding Out

In A.D. 700, a beautiful Irish Princess, Dymphna, fled to Belgium with her Confessor because of the incestuous advances of her father. Her father overtook them in the little Flemish community of Gheel not far from Antwerp and decapitated her.

The people of Gheel, disturbed and mystified by such bizarre behaviour, preserved Dymphna's body. Over a period, her remains became invested with magical significance for people suffering from mental illness. Dymphna became a saint and Gheel a place of pilgrimage for the mentally sick.

A healing ritual developed in which the patient, with a clay amulet engraved with some letters of Dymphna's name hung about the neck, crept on hands and knees under the shrine containing the Princess's bones. The ritual was repeated on a number of days and the whole process could be carried out as many times as the patient or relatives wished.

The church containing the remains of the saint had a number of annexes for housing pilgrims during their stay. These soon became inadequate and the pious people of Gheel started taking the pilgrims into their homes.

This is the legend behind the first boarding-out scheme for psychiatric patients (Dumont and Aldrich, 1962). Over the years patients travelled to Gheel from all over Belgium and Holland and from as far away as New Zealand and the United States of America. The cure ritual became less important and the object of going to Gheel was more to find asylum in a free and normal community when the only other choice was life in a prison-like mental institution.

In 1860, 800 patients were living and working with

families in the community. By 1940 the number had risen to 3,700. Since then there has been a steady decrease owing to changes in official policy and administration. Recently there has been some revitalization and there is hope that the scheme will survive. For it not to survive would be a tragedy, since boarding out and finding normal homes for those who are unable to return to a fully independent life outside hospital are now looked upon as an important part of rehabilitating psychiatric patients.

The first family care programme was started in the United States in Massachusetts in 1855. In Britain, subnormal children and adults have been boarded out for many years, but it is only since the last war that schemes for elderly and psychiatric patients have really been developed. Some very successful projects have been carried out in Plymouth and Exeter for old people (National Corporation for the Care of Old People, 1960, National Old People's Welfare Council, 1960), while Exvale Hospital, Exeter, operates a flourishing scheme for psychiatric patients (Helen Slater, 1964).

Boarding out can play three main roles in the complex of psychiatric care. It can be a stepping stone between hospital and full independence in the community. In many cases, to return home following recovery is inadvisable, particularly for one group of schizophrenics. Boarding out can be either a stepping stone or a more permanent solution to these patients' accommodation problems. Many elderly patients in psychiatric hospitals have lost their homes and relatives. This may be the result of spending too many years in hospital or the rapid destruction of their place in the community following admission in old age. For these, boarding out can offer a chance of returning to the community and to a more normal life. Again, this may be a permanent solution or a step towards finding new homes of their own and the added independence this carries. A third important function of boarding out is the prevention of admission or re-admission to hospital. Occasionally a patient being dealt with on an out-patient or day-patient basis loses his home or is rejected by his family. Without boarding out, the only solution may be admission to hospital with all the dangers this can still entail.

BOARDING OUT FROM SEVERALLS

Since 1960, large numbers of long-stay patients have been discharged from Severalls. This was the result of the dramatic changes in care and atmosphere produced by the physician superintendent and the medical and nursing staff. One result of this depletion in long-stay patients was that the patients remaining in the psychogeriatric unit posed serious problems of rehabilitation and re-settlement. The less problematic patients had been discharged, leaving the most difficult, and what some considered hopeless, cases behind. The majority had no homes or interested families and were completely unfamiliar with the changed world outside. Many members of staff considered that it would be better if they spent the rest of their days in hospital and viewed any move to re-establish them in the community as unkind and inhumane.

In spite of these difficulties and some personal doubts, I persuaded a few staff members that a boarding-out scheme could work and would help some patients to a better life. Helen Slater's work with boarding out at Exvale Hospital and the reports of other workers in Britain convinced one unit social worker that it could be done and the Severalls scheme was launched in December 1963. Meetings were held to which various voluntary and official organizations were invited. This resulted in much free publicity in the local papers and some in the nationals, but there was little response from the public. One elderly lady offered the use of a cottage she owned, but she had not seen the papers and it was a coincidence that she approached the hospital at this time. She had taken in younger patients as lodgers, knew there were patients in the hospital who were there only because they had nowhere to live, and finding her next-door cottage vacant, thought it could be used for these patients. Living a rather lonely life, she also hoped for company.

Encouraged by the success of others, advertising in the 'Accommodation Wanted' and 'Personal' columns of local papers was tried. Some examples of the advertisements used are:

Foster homes wanted for elderly persons under the Severalls Hospital scheme of boarding out. Apply to Mrs. J. V. Graham, Social Worker, Severalls Hospital, Colchester.

Wanted, offers of a home for a lady aged 68 years, able to care for herself but still under care of hospital as weekly day patient.

Elderly lady, able to look after herself and now only in hospital because she has no home, wants board with accommodation under hospital boarding-out scheme £4 to £5.

It is considered important to make clear in the advertisement that the patients are at Severalls and give the name of a specific person to communicate with in the hospital. This approach met with success and has continued to be used up to the present.

When anyone replies to an advertisement she is visited by the unit social worker responsible for operating the scheme, who assesses the situation, and if it appears suitable she is invited to the hospital to meet some of the patients who are waiting to be boarded out. At this stage the potential hostess is given a specially prepared leaflet describing the boarding-out scheme and giving advice on money and what to do in emergencies, which include physical sickness and death. The latter subject is mentioned because hostesses are often anxious about what will happen if the patient dies and few know that if they make arrangements for the funeral they can be held responsible for payment.

It is preferred that a hostess and the patient get to know each other by exchange of visits before the patient finally leaves the hospital. Usually the patient goes for a holiday with the potential hostess before finally being discharged. In this way the patients are not disappointed if things do not work out, since it is explained that they are going for a holiday and no specific mention is made of them staying with the family permanently. If there is mutual satisfaction with the arrangement, the possibility of a more permanent stay is then discussed. Support continues after the patient is discharged. As far as possible, the social worker calls once a week in the first place and then reduces the frequency of visits if things are going satisfactorily. A number of boarded-out patients continue to attend the day hospital and it is felt that this has certain advantages. Many long-stay patients get a certain amount of support by simply coming back to the hospital and meeting their old friends.

The majority of boarded-out patients are financed by the Ministry of Social Security since they usually have no funds of their own. The hostess receives £4 to £5 and the ex-patient £1 6s. 0d. The hostess is always offered support and the assurance that the patient will be taken back into the hospital if things do not work out satisfactorily. However, it is pointed out that there may be some problems of adjustment and that it would be to the patient's disadvantage if the hostess gave up too quickly. The social worker, during her visits, not only assesses the state of the patient and discusses the patient's problems, but also helps and guides the hostess. She persuades and encourages the hostess to allow as much independence as possible to the ex-patient, allowing him to handle his own money, possess a rent book and involve himself in community activities.

In the early stages of the scheme, it was realized that the ordinary rehabilitation programmes in the unit were not sufficient for the patients being boarded out. Because of this a special mixed rehabilitation ward was set up in the unit. Patients who were possibly suitable for boarding out were transferred to this ward for final assessment and intensive rehabilitation. The ward sister became very much interested and keen on boarding out and has played a very important and active part in making the scheme successful. She encourages the patients to buy their own clothes, do their own shopping and do some cooking and other household duties in the Household Management Unit. She also visits them after they have left hospital and invites hostesses to the ward at regular intervals for tea-parties. This has resulted in the development of a group spirit among both the hostesses and the patients. Families who board out patients are also invited to the monthly relatives' conference held in the unit. Some of the hostesses play a very active part in the group discussions at these meetings and are often able to offer advice and support to families who are caring for their own elderly relatives who attend the day hospital.

Between 1963 and 1967, seventy-nine patients were boarded out (fifty-nine women, twenty men). Their ages ranged from 55 to 80 and their length of stay in hospital before leaving from two to fifty-two years. Six died, eight were transferred to welfare homes, private homes or their own home and ten returned to hospital, leaving fifty-five still boarded out in 1967. Diagnostic categories have included dementia, depression, schizophrenia, paraphrenia, personality disorders and subnormality. No patient boarded out has caused any trouble or disturbance in the community and there has been no serious complaint from hostesses. Some hostesses complained of minor idiosyncrasies, usually because they considered that the hospital staff should be informed, or wanted to know if any change in treatment or management was necessary.

The first attempt at boarding out undertaken by the unit was rather atypical and involved the old lady and her cottage referred to before.

THE COTTAGE

The owner offered the cottage next to her own for use by the unit to accommodate three ladies. The unit's social worker specifically responsible for boarding out visited, and was not impressed. Situated on a busy road, old and four-roomed, it had few refinements. The front door opened into the living-room, the back door into the kitchen, a narrow, dark staircase without handrail led up to one single and one double bedroom and there was no bath or bathroom. The rooms were clean but sparsely furnished, the kitchen containing an antiquated electric cooker but no means of heating water except in a kettle. Some light switches were loose. A water closet at the end of a narrow back garden was approached by way of two, possibly dangerous, steps. The front and back doors fitted badly, improving ventilation but decreasing comfort.

The owner, Miss H., was 74 years old, short, thin, intelligent, obviously lonely and apparently with few interests. She had been brought up in an orphanage, spending most of her life as a cook in various hotels, schools and private houses. Her only capital was her property and her income an old age pension, so she could afford little for improving the cottage.

Normally, great care must be taken when selecting and matching patients for boarding out. They should be introduced to their new home over a period, so ensuring as far as possible mutual acceptance before committing either side. This procedure could not be applied since Miss H.

required tenants quickly. She was short of money, lonely, unoccupied and, it was believed, in danger of slipping into the misery and hopelessness of solitary old age.

There were many doubts about the suitability of the accommodation; there were a host of structural disadvantages, the furnishings and equipment were inadequate and there was little money available to pay for improvements. Hospital patients are used to warmth, comfortable beds, abundant hot water, easy access to toilets and readily available entertainment. The cottage would be relatively cold, the beds less comfortable, hot water difficult to produce, the toilet was outside and there was no radio or television. It was doubted if this would be boarding out in the sense of a patient leaving hospital for a real home where she would be accepted and given a place. It appeared that the ladies would leave hospital for accommodation next door to the real home and possibly become more isolated than in hospital, with the danger of Miss H. playing the part of the old-type psychiatric nurse, attending to their physical needs, but ignoring their emotional wants.

The Patients

With the doubts remaining, plans were nevertheless made to improve the cottage and three patients were selected:

Mrs L. K., a widow of 74, who had been in hospital for forty-one years. Admitted because of hypomania, her illness had taken a variable course, but she had been well enough to leave hospital for some years, remaining only because she had nowhere to live. A son who had been a patient in Severalls lived in lodgings in Colchester, but was unable to help. At the time of selection she was a cheerful institutionalized old lady who otherwise showed little evidence of mental illness.

Mrs D. J., a widow of 70, admitted twenty-four years previously because of depression. During her stay in hospital she had improved, but remained over-quiet and spoke only when spoken to. She had worked for many years in the sewing room, had made few friends and was never visited.

Mrs A. W., a 64-year-old widow with agitated depression who had been in hospital for six years, having been admitted on two previous occasions between 1945 and 1958. She had made a good recovery but remained in hospital because of accommodation difficulties. A brother and sister visited but could not help. At the time of selection she was cheerful but unsure of herself and was becoming dependent on the hospital.

Moving In

It was possible with the aid of the Women's Voluntary Service and other voluntary help to make some improvements to the cottage. A handrail was fitted for the stairs, light switches repaired and sited nearer the beds for night use, a fast boiling-ring substituted for an old hot-plate on the cooker and curtains fitted to the doors to reduce draughts. Two single beds replaced a double bed in the larger bedroom and the general comfort was enhanced by the addition of extra blankets, pillows, cushions, and chair covers.

Following completion of these improvements, the patients moved in. While in hospital they had all saved a little money which was now placed in individual Post Office Savings Bank Accounts. Each received £4 16s. 0d. from the old National Assistance Board, out of which they paid £3 15s. 0d. rent. The rent included full board, Miss H. buying food and preparing all their meals. Because there was no bath, arrangements were made for the patients to attend the day hospital at Severalls each week. Here they would be able to have a bath, see their friends and be seen by a doctor if necessary. The unit Social Worker visited the cottage weekly to ensure that the National Assistance Board money was being collected, the rent paid and that everything was running smoothly.

Development Into a Family

During the first few weeks some difficulties became apparent. The patients missed the radio and television, had few visitors and complained of boredom. Miss H. became over-protective and anxious. She treated Mrs L.K. as a favourite, but complained of Mrs A.W. because she was careless and of Mrs D.J. because she was silent.

It was possible to solve most of these problems. The Rotary Club supplied a radio and visitors were encouraged, visits being made by hospital staff, the local vicar, patients' relatives and members of the Women's Voluntary Service. When the ladies visited the day hospital it was possible to see Miss H. alone so that she could voice her fears, seek advice and generally discuss her problems.

In time all four began to accept each other's difficulties and limitations. Household duties were more evenly distributed, Miss H. spent more time with her boarders, eating all her meals with them and spending most of her evenings in their company. Better contact was made with the outside world; regular visits were made to the shops and they became active members of the local old people's club, attending meetings regularly and going on a number of day trips during the summer.

After six months, a family group developed, the two cottages became one functional unit and there was little doubt that all four had benefited. Miss H. was no longer lonely, she had developed an interest in life and lost much of her anxiety. Perhaps the feelings of the three ex-patients were expressed by Mrs L.K., when she said that her greatest pleasure was to have a key to open her own door and to be able to ask visitors in to tea.

OTHER ILLUSTRATIVE CASES

The following three examples of boarding out are more typical of the scheme, in that the patients became members of pre-existing families.

Miss B. W., aged 61. In the course of five years she had eight admissions to hospital because of depression. On the last occasion her unmarried brother refused to have her back and the whole family were against her leaving hospital again. In spite of this opposition it was possible to place her in her own familiar district with a middle-aged married couple and their daughter. In 1967 she had been boarded out for three years, but had required two short admissions for relapses. By this time her improvement was such that she was able to visit her family for week-ends without causing distress either to them or herself. She continues to be seen regularly every two to four weeks in the day hospital for supportive treatment.

Mr E. P., aged 79. Originally admitted to an institution in 1909 because of subnormality, he was transferred to Severalls in 1913 when the hospital was opened. He was described in the notes at that time as feeble minded, emotionally unstable and entirely dependent on the hospital. For many years he worked in the printer's shop until he was transferred to the psychogeriatric unit because of age. In August 1965 he was considered suitable for boarding out since his family would have nothing to do with him. The social worker concerned went to a great deal of trouble to find a suitable place for him. Success finally resulted from seeing an advertisement on the notice board of a shop. The home consisted of an elderly couple of Salvationists. Mr E.P. settled in very quickly and was adamant that he had no wish to return to hospital. Readmission has not been necessary.

Mr W. P., aged 78. When he was 22 he murdered his wife and was sentenced to death. He was reprieved and sent to a hospital for the criminally insane. In 1963 he was transferred to the psychogeriatric unit at Severalls because it was no longer considered necessary to keep him in a semi-penal institution. On admission he was considered a suitable case for boarding out, but because of his criminal record much thought was given to his placing. Tentative inquiries were made to religious bodies in the town but no offers were forthcoming. Finally careful inquiries were made of a couple known to the social worker, Mr and Mrs Y. Mrs Y. had been in charge of an elderly people's residential home but had given this up because of ill health. Knowing the whole story, they took Mr. W. P. into their home on a holiday basis, having invited him to the house for tea on a number of occasions. He settled in and so endeared himself to the host and hostess that he was discharged after being with them for two weeks. Unfortunately, after being out for only five months he developed acute retention of urine and died in the local general hospital.

Workers in the unit consider that the boarding-out scheme has been fairly successful and this has been confirmed by patients, relatives and hosts and hostesses.

Fears that patients who had spent long periods in hospital would not settle in the community and would be unhappy were completely unfounded. The findings of other workers in this field have in part been confirmed. Contrary to expectation, older patients and patients who had been in hospital for ten or more years have tended to make the best adjustment. Some workers have suggested that patients with a history of unpredictable or erratic behaviour do badly when boarded out. This has not been confirmed. Patients with histories of erratic behaviour have been boarded out and have not presented any problem. Behaviour in hospital is not a reliable measure of what behaviour might be like in a normal home. The authoritarian, restrictive atmosphere still present in some wards in even very good hospitals may produce disturbed behaviour in patients who are in fact normal, and will not put up with petty restrictions and bossy attitudes.

Whatever the degree to which they have become adjusted, boarded-out patients have become more alive and active and more interested in their surroundings, while their expression and bearing has changed markedly for the better.

There have been more applications from would-be hosts from rural than from urban areas, which is in keeping with other workers' findings in Britain. It may be that different methods for finding homes are necessary in urban districts. When it has been possible to persuade councils to allow their tenants to take in patients, a new source of urban homes has been revealed.

At the beginning it was thought that some people might apply to have a patient for their own benefit, wanting them as cheap baby-sitters or housekeepers. There have been applications from this group, but it has been remarkably easy to pick out those who were unsuitably motivated. In the early days of the project an application for a 'grandmother' was received from Heidelberg. The letter appeared suspicious and was suggestive of someone trying to obtain cheap help. It was obviously impossible to board someone out in Germany even if the family were genuine in their desire to help the elderly. The Heidelberg family were referred to a German social agency who discovered they were themselves in need of social, if not psychiatric, help.

The small remuneration for boarding-out accommodation has tended to discourage ill-motivated applicants. The majority of people interested in the scheme have been middle-aged or elderly, many being widows. There have been remarkably few requests from young people.

Some of the hostesses have benefited almost as much from having a patient living with them as the patient has benefited from being in the community. The patient has combated their loneliness, introduced a new interest in their lives and widened the range of their friends.

Some families required more help and support than others and this occasionally presented difficulties, because the unit social worker had many other commitments to the unit. If it had been possible to employ a social worker full-time on boarding out, the greater involvement would have resulted in homes being used about which there were some doubts. It might also have been possible to have tapped other sources of accommodation by canvassing private houses and by the systematic search of shop notice boards. In fact one patient found a home when the social worker used this method, but unfortunately it could not be repeated because it was too time consuming.

Accommodation offered should not be too quickly dismissed as inadequate or unsuitable. Reasonable standards of physical comfort are important but should not be the only criteria. The cottage described is an example of accommodation where the apparent physical comfort was much less than that provided by the hospital, yet there was little doubt where the three ladies preferred to be.

Boarding out has not been looked upon as an end in itself, even for the group of elderly patients dealt with. Some patients have moved on to a much more independent life, while others have returned to their families.

It would appear that there are large numbers of old people in hospitals throughout the country who could end their lives back in the community in happier circumstances if more use were made of boarding out. To make a boarding-out scheme work, it is essential that a well-organized rehabilitation programme is mounted in the hospital. The staff involved in the programme need to be in close communication with the social worker who is dealing with boarding out, and with the host families, both before and after the patient leaves hospital. The Severalls scheme has been fortunate in having one social worker who put a considerable amount of energy and interest into the project and became personally involved in its success or failure. Much of her spare time is spent in dealing with the problems of patients and hostesses. The other unit social worker, though not directly responsible for the scheme, did much to make it successful and also spends her spare time helping with the service and finding accommodation.

Psychotherapeutic guidance has been necessary for staff, hostesses, hosts and patients. Therapy and advice provided has had to be such that there is the minimum interference with the family structures that are developing. Formal, individual and group psychotherapy has played a part, but the most important guidance has occurred at staff meetings, relatives' conferences and during informal meetings between everyone involved. Staff fears and anxieties have to be brought into the open and freely discussed before hosts and patients can be helped. Allowance must be made for popular misconceptions of mental illness and old age when dealing with both staff and hosts. On the whole the patients have presented the least problems and made the best adjustments.

References

Boarding Out of Old People, National Corporation for the Care of Old People, London, 1960.

Boarding Out Schemes for Elderly People, National Old People's Welfare Council, London, 1960.

Dumont, M. P., and Aldrich, C. K., 'Family care after 1000 Years – a crisis in the tradition of Saint Dymphna', *American Journal of Psychiatry*, August 1962, pp. 116–21.

Slater, Helen, 'The Community helps the Discharged Long-Stay Patient', *Case Conference* January 1964, pp. 109–12.

10 | Hospital, Family and Community

There are many divergent views of the origins of psychiatric illness. Some psychiatrists consider the life experience of the patient all-important, some emphasize inheritance, while others ignore everything except the present clinical picture. Whatever view is held, it is important to know something about the family and community situation and attempt to involve them in therapy. The majority of patients have relatives and friends and live or have lived in communities. Even long-stay inmates of institutions may have living relatives, a friend from the past, or some other slender connexion with the community in which they once lived. A better understanding of the total situation that leads to a request for treatment or admission should make any attempt to re-establish the patient in the community more effective. Patients in hospital are more likely to respond to treatment if they maintain contact with relatives and friends and keep in touch with the outside world. Lack of these contacts is likely to produce withdrawal and the development of institutional neurosis. The successful maintenance of a patient in the community or his resettlement after admission is always dependent on the attitudes of family, friends and neighbours.

In spite of these factors and continued teaching on the subject, some hospital staff show little interest in relatives and in any other contacts patients may have with the community. In the extreme situation, patients are treated in almost complete isolation from reality. Little information is obtained about the home situation, relatives are seen only if they ask for an interview and the patient may be discharged without anyone outside the hospital who may be concerned being consulted or informed. Some doctors consider relatives to be a source of trouble and irritation, expressing their attitude in terms such as, 'Do I have to see the relatives, Sister?' and, 'Not those relatives again.'

Nursing staff are usually forced into a closer relationship than doctors with relatives and other visitors, but how these relationships develop depends on the attitude of the medical staff and the general atmosphere in the hospital. If the administrative and therapeutic structure encourages remoteness between staff and patients, relatives will feel unwelcome and their conversations with staff will be inhibited and mutually uninformative.

In authoritarian hospitals, where visiting is restricted to a few hours per week, relatives who wish to see a doctor may be lined up like army defaulters outside his office and seen so rapidly that there is hardly time for even the normal greetings that occur when people meet. Friends may be told that they cannot be given information because they are not relatives, and relatives themselves may be fobbed off with vague, disquieting statements. These are the conditions that produce difficult relatives. Some people do tend to be aggressive and awkward in their relationships with others but experience indicates that the majority of so-called difficult relatives do not belong to this rather small group. They become difficult because of staff attitudes. Many doctors and nurses have met relatives said to be difficult by others and found this to be untrue. Aggressive behaviour changes in the face of kindness and being treated like an intelligent adult.

The majority of psychiatrists and geriatricians discovered long ago that the successful treatment of their patients depended on involving the family and sometimes the community in the therapeutic situation. Family and community understanding and interest had to be generated if many of their patients were to be maintained or re-established in society. Unfortunately, this knowledge does not necessarily lead to the development of better relationships. Visitors to a hospital are influenced and affected by a great variety of staff. Telephonists, receptionists, porters, clerks, a whole range of administrators, nurses, social workers, occupational therapists, doctors, engineers, kitchen workers, cleaners and management committee members can all play a part in creating a right or wrong impression of the hospital. A bossy porter brushing aside a relative's request for information not only gives a bad impression of the hospital but may sow the seed of further conflict. Annoyed by his attitude, the relative may be aggressive when seeing the ward doctor or nurse, and a chain reaction may occur. The ward doctor or nurse complain to their seniors who, expecting trouble, find it when they meet the disgruntled relative – and another relative is branded as difficult.

The treatment of patients does not depend on a doctor and a few nurses, but involves everyone in the hospital and must be influenced by the quality of inter-personal relationships within the institution.

Provided the hospital is run on progressive lines, a number of methods can be used to involve the family and stimulate community interest and concern. Access to the hospital should be easy, so that relatives and friends can come and go with the minimum of restriction. Members of the public may be encouraged to visit the hospital if Open Days are organized and it is made known that visitors are always welcomed. Talks and films to community groups may provide some information but their main object should be an introduction to visiting the hospital. One visit can do more to change the stereotype of what a mental hospital is like than a thousand lectures. Relatives and those closely involved with the patient should be seen as frequently as necessary by the appropriate doctor, social worker or nurse. Relatives may be involved in group therapy, either with patients or in a separate relatives' group. At Severalls a relatives' group has been developed that operates in association with individual interviews and involvement in ward activities.

THE RELATIVES' CONFERENCE

There have been a number of accounts of relatives' conferences in psychiatric hospitals in Canada and the U.S.A. In Britain the number reported has been small. In 1964, M. B. Hawker described relatives' meetings held in the geriatric unit of Edgware General Hospital. Following this article, the staff of the psychogeriatric unit at Severalls became interested. Some staff members visited Edgware General Hospital and meetings were started at Severalls in August 1964. It was at first hoped to hold the meetings outside the hospital in Colchester, so as to reduce transport difficulties for relatives. This was not possible, which was fortunate, because it would have meant a diminished contact with the hospital. The first meeting was held in the hospital committee room – a venue with a number of disadvantages. The atmosphere was formal, there was little room for freedom of movement and it seemed far away from patients and the realities of hospital life. The next and subsequent meetings were held in the unit day hospital which was common ground for relatives and patients and there was ample space for demonstrations, films and exhibitions.

The meetings take place on the last Monday in each month and start at approximately 7 p.m. A programme is sent to all relatives and anyone else who may be or should be interested, including hospital and local authority staff, voluntary organizations and people interested in the problems of the elderly. The programme is usually sent out a week before the meeting, and so acts as a reminder.

The meetings are as informal as possible, but usually

start with an organized event. This might be a lecture, film or demonstrations and is usually the result of requests by relatives at previous meetings. Lectures have been given by unit doctors, nurses, social workers and outside speakers, subjects ranging from housing for the elderly to causes of confusional states. Demonstrations are usually of methods for dealing with physical disabilities. An exhibition of aids for the disabled and information on diet and services for the elderly are features of each meeting.

The organized part of the meeting is followed by refreshments. It is here that the most important part of the proceedings starts. The exchange of social pleasantries develops into discussion and before long mutual problems relating to patients are being freely discussed. Doubts and grievances are brought into the open, ideas are swapped and personal misunderstandings uncovered. Relatives learn that their problems are not unique. The staff come to realize that the problems presented by patients at home are different from those in hospital, while relatives learn of the effect of the hospital on the patient.

Staff have obtained important information about individual patients during these discussions. This has occurred in a number of different ways. Some relatives have been better able to mention difficulties and describe the behavioural problems of the patient in the relaxed atmosphere of the conference. Others have found it easier to discuss their problems and anxieties when these same problems and anxieties have already been described by the more articulate.

Quite frequently people attending the meetings have mentioned an old person in the community who they have considered to be in need of help. The unit staff always investigate these cases and have usually been able to provide help, particularly by organizing community care or attendance at the day hospital.

Ideas for improving the organization of the unit and subjects for research have also been put forward by relatives and others who attend the meetings. These have included the method for keeping general practitioners and the family informed of changes in clinical condition and treatment already mentioned, an investigation into the nutritional state of new day patients compared to those who had attended for a prolonged period and ways of publicizing the work of the unit by keeping local newspapers informed of what was happening in the hospital.

In one discussion lack of certain equipment for physiotherapy and occupational therapy was mentioned. Following this meeting, a group of relatives organized a social in a local village and raised sufficient money to purchase the necessary equipment.

Some relatives appear to benefit from the support given by the meetings. Some have struck up new friendships and so combated their own loneliness and isolation. A few continue to attend after the patient has died or ceased to be connected with the hospital. This is never discouraged since they appear to find it beneficial to attend and are usually able to make a contribution to the group.

During the period in which conferences have been held, the average attendance at each meeting has been twenty relatives, plus staff and other visitors. One reason that the numbers have been relatively small is the nature and size of the hospital's catchment area. Relatives may have to travel long distances and, because the area is mainly rural, public transport is often inadequate. When it has been possible to supply transport for some families, the numbers have increased and many relatives have said they would attend if transport of some kind were available. Attempts have been made to organize a voluntary car service. This has so far been unsuccessful, but the attempts continue.

Staff have often suggested that the meetings were not attracting the relatives who would most benefit from attending. This is possibly true, but difficult to remedy. Attempts are always being made to improve the quality of the programme and increase its appeal. Staff and patients are encouraged to use their persuasive abilities, and information about meetings is sent out regularly to all relatives, whether they attend or not.

Relatives who do attend regularly appear to profit from the experience and the hospital has also gained from holding the meetings. Some relatives have developed an interest in the day hospital, involving themselves in its social activities, while others go out of their way to spread information about the hospital in the community. Staff claim that they learn from this type of association with relatives and believe that the patients benefit from the relatives' greater understanding of their problems.

Experience of relatives' meetings over a period of two and a half years indicates that they can play a useful part in any psychogeriatric service. The experience of others, including the staff of the geriatric unit of Edgware General Hospital and two psychiatric hospitals in Britain, suggests that they have a role in general psychiatry and geriatric practice. There do not appear to be any published papers on such meetings in general hospitals for the relatives of patients with medical or surgical illness. It may be claimed that they are not appropriate in this setting since medical and surgical patients are under hospital care for only comparatively short periods and that on this account relatives' opinions and cooperation are not important. This is not true. Very many patients who are treated in general and specialized medical and surgical departments remain under some type of hospital care for long periods. Examples are patients with chronic respiratory and cardiac disease, diabetes mellitus, collagen diseases and various neurological disorders. These patients often have interested relatives, usually have social difficulties and, at least in part, depend on a satisfactory community response to their disability. Doubts and misunderstandings between general hospital staff and relatives are not uncommon. Relatives' meetings in the general hospital may have similar effects to those held at Severalls and at other psychiatric hospitals. In these institutions doubts and misunderstandings have not vanished, but do appear to have been reduced. The free exchange of views is the only antidote at present available for a lack of understanding between different groups.

The relatives' meetings, as well as having a therapeutic function, also help to reduce the gap between hospital and community. At Severalls, a number of other methods have been used to achieve this objective, including greater freedom for patients, unrestricted visiting, visits by community groups to the hospital, open days, lectures, films, the use of mass media propaganda and – perhaps most important – individual efforts by the staff in their everyday contact with people from outside the hospital. The importance of staff attitudes to relatives and visitors has been mentioned. The employment of specially selected telephonists and receptionists has done much to improve the quality of the visitors' first encounter with the hospital. Many people make their first contact by telephone. A pleasant greeting from the telephonist can be the foundation of a good relationship. Kindly receptionists make visitors feel at ease, and help to reduce the sense of perplexity common on first visiting a large strange institution. The attitudes of the medical and nursing staff have been slowly changed by example, exhortation and the therapeutic effect of the various staff and patient/staff meetings. Meetings tend to be confined to patients, doctors, nurses, social workers and occupational therapists. At some psychiatric hospitals other staff are involved, including porters. The latter are often a significant link between visitors and hospital staff, and their participation in meetings is as useful as that of any other staff.

Over a period, the outside community's image of Severalls has improved. This has been part of a gradual change in the relationship between psychiatric hospitals and society in Britain, but further change is necessary before old fears and misconceptions disappear, and even so each change can bring further problems. A recent survey at Severalls revealed one previously unknown disadvantage of unrestricted visiting. Under the previous system, visiting was allowed only between specific times on specific days. Doctors knew when visitors would be in the hospital and could make themselves available for interviews. With unrestricted visiting, visitors come at any time and, if they want to see the ward sister or doctor, they may find them absent or unavailable. Appointments can be made but this involves another visit to the hospital, often from a considerable distance. At present this problem is being investigated and possible solutions are being tested out. The simple expedient of writing for an appointment before a visit does not solve the problem, because the need to see a doctor can often arise urgently.

The proper practice of psychiatry should entail the treatment of the patient and family in the setting of the community. What has been described is an attempt at a few faltering steps in the direction of this ideal.

Reference

Hawker, M. B., 'The Relatives' Conference', *Lancet*, 16 May 1964. p. 1,098.

11 | Conclusions

The psychogeriatric service developed at Severalls has been described in some detail. It is an example of one administrative structure catering for one group of old people, but it does illustrate the kind of geriatric care being evolved in Britain.

The problems of ageing and the elderly are of interest to a large number of workers in varied disciplines. Sociologists, architects, occupational therapists, physiotherapists, general physicians, geriatricians, pathologists, physiologists, psychoanalysts, eclectic psychiatrists, surgeons, psychologists and biochemists are all making contributions. The report of a symposium on 'Psychiatric Disorders of the Aged' held by the World Psychiatric Association in 1965 illustrates some of the many different approaches to the problems of old people with mental illness.

The knowledge that is accumulating should benefit the elderly, but can do so only if it is readily available to the personnel involved in their treatment, care and support. To make this possible, geriatric services must be organized in such a way that they are receptive to new ideas and provide a milieu in which knowledge can easily be spread to all grades of workers in the service. The Severalls project is an attempt to produce such an organization, which also provides a complex of services to deal with the problems of today and prepare for the problems of tomorrow. A complex of services is necessary, since different problems require different solutions, and failure to provide this complex usually means inadequate care. The provisions at Severalls are not ideal and many problems remain unsolved and some unidentified; but it has been possible to evolve a system which maintains a large number of old people fairly successfully in the community, reduces the number of in-patients and makes reasonably efficient use of limited resources of money and manpower.

It has been said that lack of money should not be used as an excuse for doing nothing. This does not mean that the Health Service does not require more money. There is urgent need for a much more extensive rebuilding programme to replace the poorly designed, crumbling ruins that masquerade as hospitals. This money may finally become available if there is sufficient public pressure and a willingness to pay. For the present, there seems little likelihood of more money being provided immediately and, if it were, staff shortages would still remain the most important difficulty. Good care can be provided in a slum and poor care in a palace. An efficient service for the elderly can be developed with the present facilities, provided someone in each area commits himself to its organization, and utilizes techniques that result in other staff becoming involved and committed. These include breaking down narrow concepts of role, the use of regular staff meetings where information can be exchanged, fears and anxieties ventilated and an opportunity provided for everyone to contribute, coupled with an organization which allows staff to implement their own ideas and be responsible for them.

Within the present Health Service structure, it would seem that it should be a doctor who takes on this role, but this may not necessarily be so in the future. A very efficient, progressive psychogeriatric unit in the U.S.A. has been developed and organized by a trained social worker. Many nurses, administrators, psychologists, social workers and other non-medical staff have qualities that make them more able to create and develop a clinical service than a doctor appointed because of narrow specialized medical skills. The present administrative structure of the Health Service makes doctors cling to their privileges and authority. They rightly believe that, once they relinquish what authority they have, others will take over and make decisions relating to patient care without their advice and perhaps against their wishes.

If it were possible to change the administrative organization so that something similar to a therapeutic community developed, these fears might become less, and it should then be possible to utilize to the best advantage the skills of all grades of personnel. Under these conditions, if there were freedom to work together, and narrow concepts of role and status disappeared, staff with administrative flair and personalities that inspire confidence could contribute to organize a service regardless of their professional label.

The expression 'therapeutic community' means different things to different people, but it is usually applied to a method of treatment in psychiatry. In bare outline, a therapeutic community is one in which patients and staff work and live together with the fewest regulations and the maximum freedom of expression. Persuasion and argument replace commands and demands, while mutual understanding and tolerance are fostered in both staff and patients. Decisions are arrived at by democratic means and no one is allowed to employ professional status as a substitute for reasoned argument.

Perhaps this is an ideal, but some hospitals at least try to operate along these lines. There is strong and vocal opposition to the concept. Some psychiatrists and nurses claim that patients with psychiatric illnesses require discipline and need to be told what to do and how to do it. Others may say that this type of treatment may be humanitarian and even effective, but that it does not prepare patients for the realities of life outside hospital. Apart from clinical arguments for and against, it does appear that staff work more efficiently

and provide a better service if these techniques are applied to them, while patients are entitled to have opinions
and should not be ordered about like prisoners. It should be
remembered that patients are people who are using a service
paid for by themselves or their families. The days of Poor
Law charity have gone, and the sooner some doctors, nurses
and administrators realize this, the sooner will all types of
patients begin to receive the kind of care they deserve and
are entitled to have.

Many nurses and other hospital personnel have authoritarian personality traits, while others are cold and remote.
Nurses and doctors are not all kindly and tolerant. In spite
of this, it is possible to produce a service that is tolerant,
understanding and sympathetic in the manner it deals with
patients. When the administrative and therapeutic atmosphere is favourable to these attitudes, people tend to con-
form to the pattern. It appears that, in general, individual
attitudes tend to mirror the attitudes of the institution.

The elderly are entitled to sympathy and tolerance and
should be treated with dignity and human respect. For this
to be possible, geriatric and psychogeriatric services need
to function – at least in part – like a therapeutic community.

The importance of family and community in the care of
the elderly has been discussed in the last chapter. It does
appear that greater use could be made of families and community voluntary workers in the active care of old people.
At present, families share the load with the hospital to a
greater or lesser degree, depending on whether the patient is
an out-patient, day patient or being dealt with on a month-
in/month-out basis. Most families do not reject their
elderly relatives and are usually very willing to help. It should
be possible to devise a system by which relatives who are
available come into the hospital and provide practical help
with the care of their old people when hospitalization becomes necessary. There is an old people's home in north

London that operates on this principle and is in fact staffed almost entirely by the relatives of its residents, with a little help from professional staff.

Voluntary workers are extensively used by hospitals in the U.S.A. and recently a number of hospitals in Britain have been experimenting in their use. Continued staff shortages should stimulate more hospital managers into considering how voluntary workers can best be used. Experience in the U.S.A. and in Britain indicates that for a voluntary service to work in a hospital a full-time paid organizer must be employed. When this is done and the person appointed has the necessary skills and feels committed, volunteers are fairly quickly recruited and placed, with the minimum of upset to themselves or professional staff.

Many nurses and other professional hospital staff distrust and dislike voluntary workers, looking upon them as interfering 'do-gooders'. It is only possible to change these views by a programme of education, personal example and the practical demonstration of the usefulness of the extra help made available when voluntary workers are welcomed in a hospital.

Voluntary workers play an important part in community care. Any voluntary-worker organization within a hospital needs to be coordinated with existing community voluntary organizations. If this is done, communication between hospital and community should be improved and inter-change of workers becomes possible. If the paid organizer in the hospital has the right kind of skills, better use may be made of the community organizations and it should be possible for helpers to be used where they are most needed at any one time, be this in the hospital or the community.

The central figure of community medicine should be the general practitioner, yet he is often not fully involved in community services, particularly when these are based on a hospital, as at Severalls. This problem has already been briefly mentioned. The difficulties are well known. General practitioners have little time to spare and there is competition from other superficially more interesting specialities. Many of them lack knowledge or interest, owing to one-sided medical education in the past. The hospital may be physically remote from the majority of practitioners in its catchment area and hospital staff may be unhelpful, condescending and unwilling to take general practitioners into their confidence.

The solution must depend on how general practice develops. It may be that psychiatry and geriatrics will become synonymous with general practice. This would be a rational development, since the majority of patients are old, mentally ill or both. For this to happen, there will have to be radical changes in medical education. These changes should occur, since they would benefit general practice, the Health Service and society.

Today, responsibility for interesting and involving the family doctor lies with the hospital staff. It is of no use to blame doctors whose knowledge of psychiatry and geriatrics gained as students was limited to a few confusing lectures and vague remarks about community care, if they lack understanding and show little interest in these subjects. The hospital staff can take the initiative by improving their communication system and organizing training programmes. More use of the telephone, shorter but better letters and fuller discussion on domiciliary visits are improvements any hospital can make at once. Educational programmes may be difficult to organize and few practitioners may attend any lectures, demonstrations or seminars that are organized. This should not matter. To think about involving the general practitioner, to plan a programme and to influence a few may be the beginning of better understanding and increased mutual trust between hospital and family doctor service.

The organization described in this book has been evolved to deal with old people with mental illness, but it has been claimed that it could equally be used for any old person in need of help. Geriatric physicians play the major part in providing hospital services for the elderly. It could be claimed that they should take over all hospital services that deal with old people: however, this would be impossible because of the number of patients involved and the range of illness exhibited. Psychiatrists are involved in geriatrics and, being involved, must make contributions that help patients and interlock with other services. They can co-operate with geriatric physicians in a number of ways. Combined community care programmes can be developed, since many of the problems of the old in the community are the same, regardless of the actual illness they may have at one point in time. Combined day hospitals have been mentioned which, if developed, could be the centre of a unified community care programme involving geriatricians, the local-authority welfare department, voluntary organizations and the psychiatrist.

One common area of dispute between the psychiatrist and the geriatrician is the appropriate placement of a patient in hospital or his transfer from one specialist to the other. Combined assessment units where geriatrician, welfare officer and psychiatrist have access to beds and can arrive at mutual decisions about the care of the patient partially solves this problem. The major disadvantage of this type of unit is that admission takes place before treatment and future care is discussed. This means that conflict may still arise. For example, a welfare officer may admit a patient who obviously requires the services provided by a geriatrician, but the geriatrician may be unwilling to take on the case because he believes the welfare officer has destroyed any chance of the patient returning to the community by dealing clumsily with the situation before admission. One solution to this type of problem would be the employment of a standard admission procedure similar to the one used at Severalls.

Practical cooperation and help between psychiatrist and geriatrician is possible in a number of ways without changing the present system. The dementias present a problem which must involve cooperation. Present resources make it impossible for any one part of the service to deal alone with this group. The association of dementia with many other disease processes also makes the sharing of this problem inevitable. Patients with dementia can and should be catered for by any service for the elderly. The psychiatrist must, however, be responsible for those whose behaviour is disturbed, or which presents problems beyond the facilities of the other services. His advice should also be available when there is any doubt about the diagnosis. The geriatrician can help the psychiatrist with problems of organic disease and physical rehabilitation. The psychiatrist can help the geriatrician by establishing psychogeriatric units, assisting in the development of community care programmes and providing an advisory service on psychiatric matters, the prevention of institutional neurosis, staff problems, communication and the problems that arise when people work together in groups.

Many changes have occurred in the services for the elderly and many more are needed, but, before anything else is done, the general public should be asked for their opinion.

This would appear to be an obvious suggestion yet many people in the health and welfare services consider any idea of consulting patients and future patients to be unnecessary and unreasonable. Perhaps the greatest failings of the Health Service are due to 'experts' imagining they know best and not consulting the people for which the service is in fact being created. Some remedies for this defect are possible within the present administrative structure. Surveys can be carried out in the community, old people under care can be asked for their views and suggestions and therapeutic communities developed in hospitals and old people's homes. A more effective and active role in administration will only be possible when the structure of regional hospital boards and management committees is changed so that there is reasonable representation of patients and the general public, in place of the present system of members being recommended by various organizations which do not include organizations of patients and their relatives.

Many psychiatric hospitals in Britain have done a great deal to provide a service that is in tune with the patient's wants and to involve patients and relatives in its development. Unfortunately these improvements have not affected all hospitals, some have lagged behind and a few have hardly escaped from the restrictive authoritarian custodial past. Meetings, symposia, lectures, demonstrations, papers in the medical journals, articles in the popular press, advice from the Ministry of Health and complaints from the public have some effect, but do not really push many backward hospitals into the twentieth century.

The resurrection of the Board of Control or the creation of some other authoritarian body that would push and cajole backward hospitals is not the answer to this problem. A therapeutic community cannot be created in a hospital by authoritarian means. Each hospital has to stimulate itself, identify its own problems and attempt to solve them by allowing all grades of staff to communicate freely with each other, participate actively in the running of the hospital and develop a feeling of involvement.

One possible method of producing the required stimulation would be for the Ministry of Health to make a kind of annual clinical audit compulsory for each hospital. Every psychiatric hospital would have to complete a fairly simple questionnaire which would consist of two main parts. The first part would ask questions similar to those put forward by Russell Barton (1965) in his suggested questionnaire for measuring the effectiveness of psychiatric hospitals. Questions would cover such subjects as the provision of day hospitals, unrestricted visiting, the number of patients employed during the day, the proportion of locked to unlocked wards and the number of patients who go home at the week-end. The second part would ask questions that are considered to measure staff morale and include questions about the incidence of sickness and accidents, staff turnover and student nurse wastage. It is fairly well established that there is a direct relationship between the incidence of sickness and accidents, absenteeism, staff wastage and turnover and the level of morale in the institution being examined.

The questionnaire would require modification as ideas of good psychiatric treatment change and more is known about how morale in institutions can be measured. The results obtained from the questionnaire would be published yearly and could be made into a sort of 'league table' of hospitals. Each management committee and regional board would have to discuss the annual findings and consider in detail the reasons for the relative positions of their hospitals and the causes for this. In parallel with the audit suggested, the Ministry of Health would need to provide a skilled advisory service which would be readily available to those hospitals with a poor 'league' position which needed help to improve. It may be thought that the hospitals which are backward would pay little attention to the results of the questionnaire; however, it is more likely that these would produce sufficient stimulation of at least some members of management or staff for only good to result.

The health and welfare services will change and improve, but this will only happen if everyone who considers improvement is necessary maintains a constant pressure on the establishment at all levels of responsibility and does not accept its excuses for doing nothing.

Reference

Barton, Russell, 'Proposed scale for rating Psychiatric Hospitals', a chapter in *Psychiatric Hospital Care*, Ballière, Tindall & Cassell, 1965.

Appendix

*Leaflet describing the General Policy and
Operation of the Unit.*

The Psychogeriatric Unit, Severalls Hospital

This leaflet is intended as a guide to staff members. It briefly
outlines the general policy and operation of the unit. It should
not be looked upon as a list of unalterable rules but more as
a series of tried base lines against which innovation can occur.

ADMISSIONS

If possible all patients should be seen before admission by a
doctor from the hospital, either in an out-patient clinic, the
Day Hospital or in their own homes. If for any reason this is
not possible, they should be visited by one of our social
workers, provided the general practitioner has no objection.

The doctor or social worker should explain to the patient
and relatives the policy of the hospital, i.e. that old people are
always better in their own home and that permanent admission to hospital should be avoided whenever possible. To
achieve this object it may be only necessary to treat the patient
as a day patient, admit for a short period, or admit on a
'month-in/month-out' basis. When this policy and the reasons
behind it are explained to the patient and relatives before
admission, cooperation is the usual result and the patient's
niche in the community is maintained.

The emergency admission of an old person should always be
discouraged, provided this can be done without endangering
the patient or the generation of ill-feeling in the family or
general practitioner. An emergency admission precludes the
above procedure, sometimes results in an unnecessary admission and may make discharge difficult.

EMERGENCY SERVICE

This is fully described in 'A Psychogeriatric Domiciliary Emergency Service' and should be used whenever necessary. Most emergencies can be dealt with by a nurse and social worker. For further information about this consult Mrs Thurlow Mrs Graham (Social Workers), Sister Garrod (Day Hospital Sister), Sister Corner (Ward Sister), Mr Walker (Assistant Chief Male Nurse) or Mr Slack (Assistant Matron).

ROUTINE ON ADMISSIONS

Whenever possible a full history should be taken and examination made on admission.

If the patient cannot give a history, it should be obtained from a relative direct, or via the social worker and the inquiry form. Special note should be made of patient's income, accommodation and its tenancy, support before admission, attitude of relatives to patient and any factor operating for or against patient's ultimate discharge.

Special Investigations

These must depend on clinical findings but should always include a biochemical and bacteriological examination of urine, haemoglobin, blood urea and blood sugar (two hours after administration of 50 grams glucose).

Urinary Incontinence

See 'Urinary Incontinence in the Aged. Propantheline Bromide as an Adjunct to Treatment'.

Programme of Treatment

A programme of investigations and treatment should be formulated at this time and should include an appropriate rehabilitation programme, proposed period that the patient should remain in hospital and suggestions for after-care, e.g. day patient, 'month-in/month-out', home visits, home help, etc. It is important to make provisional plans for the patient's discharge now because it may be necessary to activate lethargic organizations, e.g. the patient's house may require cleaning and the organization of this simple task can take weeks.

If admission is on a 'month-in/month-out' basis the date of discharge should be fixed and in all cases a provisional date of discharge should be arranged always within the period of one month.

PARANOID STATES

See 'Fluphenazine Enanthate in the Treatment of Paranoid States of the Elderly'.

AFTER ADMISSION

Obviously treatment will be reviewed as necessary, but should always be reviewed one week before the discharge date. If the patient is to attend the day hospital after discharge, he or she should attend there for a few days *before* discharge to become familiar with the new surroundings and staff.

DISCHARGES

All patients for discharge are discussed at the 9.30 a.m. meeting each Thursday. Relatives should be given ample warning of a patient's discharge and after-care arrangements should be made before discharge takes place. These may include visits by a psychiatric social worker, mental welfare officer, health visitor or district nurse, home help, assistance from the welfare department with aids for the handicapped and arrangements to attend outside clubs.

THURSDAY MORNING MEETING

At this meeting all recently admitted patients are reviewed, alterations in the original programme decided and discharges arranged.

WEEKLY PROGRAMME OF MEETINGS

See attached sheet.

PATIENTS' MEETINGS

Ward doctors should arrange regular weekly patients' meetings and spend as much time as possible talking to patients on and off the ward.

DAY HOSPITAL

Day patients should be seen regularly.

At 2.0 p.m. each Friday there is a group meeting with the patients followed by a staff meeting.

BOARDING OUT

See 'An Example of Boarding out Elderly Psychiatric Patients' and 'Boarding Out Elderly Psychiatric Patients'.

Mrs Graham and Mrs Thurlow (Social Workers) are responsible for boarding out and will have all the information about it.

DENE WARD

This is a mixed ward used for the rehabilitation of long-stay patients who are considered possible for discharge home, boarding out or Part III Accommodation.

RELATIVES' CONFERENCE

Relatives' Conferences are held in the Day Hospital on the last Monday of the month at 7.0 p.m. For information please contact Mr Slack (Assistant Matron), Mrs Graham or Mrs Thurlow (Social Workers).

BED STATE

If possible there should always be two beds available in each admission ward for emergencies.

In the Service of Old Age

Timetable of Regular Meetings

MONDAY: 9.30 a.m.   Meeting for doctors, social work-
                          ers, assistant matron, assistant
                          chief male nurse, in Male Geriatric
                          Unit Headquarters.
TUESDAY: 9.30 a.m.   Meeting for doctors, social work-
                          ers, assistant matron, assistant
                          chief male nurse, in Male Geriatric
                          Unit Headquarters.
              10.30 a.m. Dr Barton's meeting with medical
                          staff.
              2.45 p.m.   Unit Meeting every third week.
WEDNESDAY: 9.00 a.m.   Meeting for doctors, social work-
                          ers, assistant matron, assistant
                          chief male nurse, in Day Hospital.
              10.30 a.m. Meeting with local authority
                          workers every fourth week.
              1.15 p.m.   Staff ward meetings on all wards.
THURSDAY: 9.30 a.m.   Unit case conference for doctors,
                          social workers, assistant matron
                          and assistant chief male nurse in
                          Male Geriatric Unit Headquarters.
FRIDAY: 9.30 a.m.   Meeting for doctors, social work-
                          ers, assistant matron, assistant
                          chief male nurse in Day Hospital.
SATURDAY: Informal staff discussion with unit
                          assistant psychiatrist.
SUNDAY: Doctors and social workers will
                          see visitors or out-patients when
                          necessary.

Relatives' Conference held on last Monday of each month at
7.0 p.m. in the Day Hospital.
Ward Sisters and Charge Nurses should organize weekly
patients' meetings at times convenient to their ward.